Feeding with Love and Good Sense:

The First 2 Years

Ellyn Satter
Dietitian and Family Therapist

Feeding with Love and Good Sense: The First 2 Years

kelcy press

ISBN 9781971847054

Developmental editor, Nancy Pekar

Part of the five-part series

Feeding with Love and Good Sense: The First Two Years
Feeding with Love and Good Sense: 18 months through 6 years
Feeding with Love and Good Sense: 6 through 13 years
Feeding with Love and Good Sense: 12 through 18 years
Feeding Yourself *with Love and Good Sense*

Show this booklet to your health care provider!

Discounted bulk purchases and PDFs of Kelcy Press books are available at https://www.ellynsatterinstitute.org/

Distributed by
Publishers Group West
819 Bancroft Way
Berkeley, CA 94710

Table of Contents

a message from Ellyn Satter

From the very first, in order to do well with feeding, focus on the *how,* not the *what.* Choosing food is important, but having a good relationship with your child around feeding is just as important. At this early stage, the *what* and *how* naturally follow right along with each other.

Feeding is parenting. In these early months and years, you spend most of your time with your child feeding. Good feeding is like a smoothly flowing conversation. Your baby asks for food and you give it, helping her to be calm and organized by paying attention to what she wants and can do. After a while—a longer while for some babies and a shorter while for others—you and your baby get on the same wavelength. Your baby was born with a longing to be understood. Your feeding in response to information coming from her lets her feel understood and therefore, loved.

When you start solid foods, toward the middle of the first year, it is the same: You go by what he tells you. He is ready for solid foods when he takes an interest in what goes on outside of just the two of you, notices your eating, sits up, and opens his mouth when he sees the food coming. You show him you understand and love him by doing it his way: feeding quickly if he wants to eat a lot in a hurry, not insisting if he doesn't want to eat.

As your child gets older, your feeding conversation changes. With your toddler, *you* start the conversation. You no longer drop everything and feed when your child asks for food. Instead, you work toward offering food at regular meals and sit-down snacks, at times you determine. Your child comes to the table, and eats—or doesn't eat. Feeding on demand, like you did when she was a baby, is no longer what she needs. As a toddler, she needs structure.

It gives you a little pang, doesn't it, thinking of your tiny and cuddly baby as an on-the-move and demanding toddler? You wouldn't be the first parent to wish you could keep your baby tiny just a bit longer! But every age and stage has its rewards and losses. As I tell my long grown-up children, "I miss you every age you have ever been. But this age is best!"

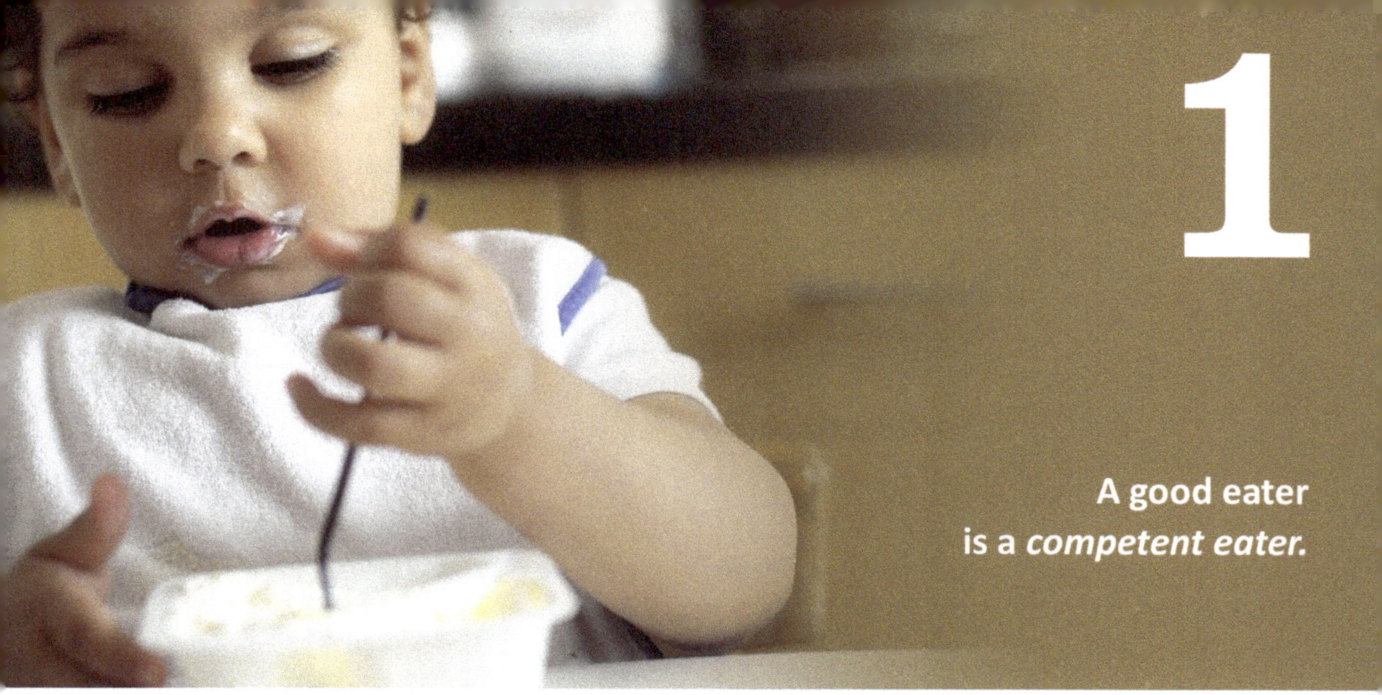

1. Where you are going with feeding

Your child's learning to be a good eater starts at birth. By 8 to 18 months, your tiny baby will be ready to join in when you have *family-friendly meals* (page 24). From the very first breast- or formula-feeding, to let your child be a good eater, focus on the *quality* of feeding rather than the *quantity* she eats.

At each step along the way, this booklet addresses your part in his learning—starting with breast- or formula-feeding, going through the steps to learn to eat grown-up food, and joining in with family meals. Step by step, your child learns to eat the food you eat and feel about eating the way you do.

A good eater is a *competent eater*

- **She feels good about eating:** Every child wants to eat and can enjoy eating if she gets the right help. Older children who are good eaters enjoy family meals—and their parents do, too.
- **She eats as much or as little as she needs:** Only she knows how much she needs. Trusting her lets her be healthy and energetic and grow up to have the body that nature intended for her.
- **She eats what you eat with only minor changes:** She is okay with being offered food she has never seen before. She can "sneak up" on new food and learn to eat it.
- **She behaves nicely at mealtime:** She picks and chooses from what you provide for the meal. She says "yes, please," and "no, thank you." She does not make a fuss.

You can raise a good eater

- Follow the division of responsibility. Doing your jobs with feeding and trusting your child to do her jobs with eating lets her feel and do best—and you, too.
- *Understand your child's development and temperament* (page 7). Feed—and parent—in the way that is right for each stage.
- Based on *what* your child can *do*, not on how *old* she is, guide your child's transition from nipple feeding through semi-solid food, then thick-and-lumpy food, to finger food at family meals.
- *Solve feeding problems* (page 33) by applying what you have learned in this booklet.

Do your jobs with feeding and let your child do her jobs with eating

- Follow the division of responsibility (next page). You do the *what, when* and *where* of *feeding* and trust your child to do the *how much* and *whether* of *eating*.
- Trust your child to grow in the way that is right for her.
- *Understand your child's development and temperament* (page 7). Feed—and parent—in the way that is right for each stage.
- *Solve feeding problems* (page 33) by applying what you have learned in this booklet.

Your child will be healthy and grow well

When you follow the division of responsibility and your child feels good about eating, she will eat as much as she needs, grow in the way that is right for her, and, over time, learn to eat a variety of food. You may feel, however, that it is your job to "get in" nutritious food or get your child to eat a certain amount and grow in a certain way. By comparison, following the division of responsibility may seem like doing nothing at all. In reality, keeping up the day-in-and-day-out of pleasant and rewarding *family friendly meals* (page 24) and *sit-down snacks* (page 31) is doing a tremendous amount. Parents say that following the division of responsibility *works* (page 6).

The division of responsibility applies to *your* special child

Every child is unusual in some way. The division of responsibility applies to all children and applies to children of all ages, birth through adolescence. The problem is that some children's characteristics and behaviors make it seem that they can't be trusted to do their part with eating. They can. With some children more than others, sticking to the division of responsibility demands steady nerves and a leap of faith. Here is help:

- The child who won't eat at mealtime (page 33).
- The "too-small" child who seemingly doesn't eat enough (page 34).
- The "too-big child" who seemingly eats too much (page 35).
- The picky eater (page 36).
- The child who doesn't eat vegetables (page 37) or drink milk (page 38).
- The child with special needs (page 39).

My toddler is a joy to feed

As a dietitian, I have studied Ellyn Satter's books and watched the *Feeding with Love and Good Sense Videos* as well so that I can counsel parents. But only since I have had a child of my own have I fully realized the importance of the division of responsibility. My husband and I look forward to mealtime with our busy toddler. My son runs eagerly to the table when we call him and we all enjoy eating together. It is so much fun to watch him eat! We let him eat whatever he wants in the meal and do not coax him to eat anything else. Our friends are amazed at how well he eats in general and how pleasant he is at the table. I am so thankful for the joy and relaxation we are able to experience at our family meals and I know it is due to the fact that we are following Ellyn Satter's philosophy—we do our jobs and we let him do his.

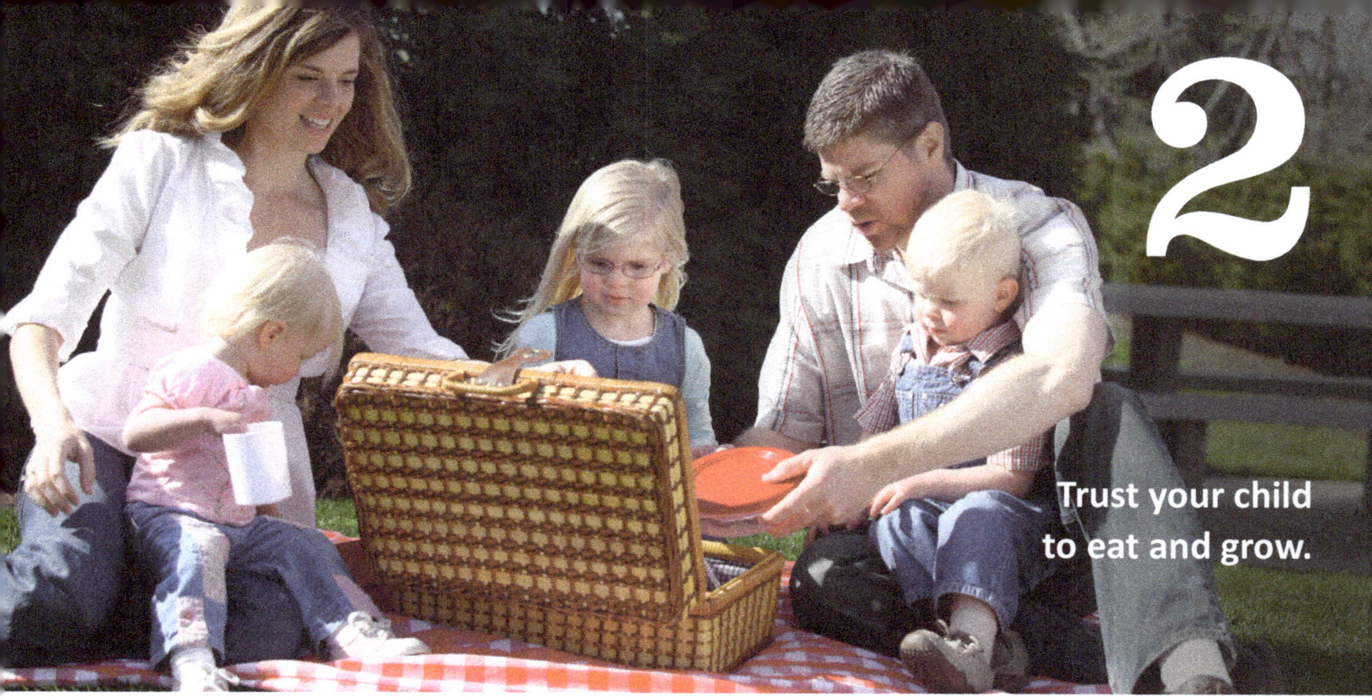

2. Follow the division of responsibility

The best way to feed your child—no matter her age—is to follow the division of responsibility. As a parent, you provide *structure, support,* and *opportunities to learn*. Your child chooses *how much* and *whether to* eat from what you provide. When you do your jobs with feeding, your child will do her jobs with eating.

The division of responsibility for infants

- You are responsible for *what* to feed your child.
- Your child is responsible for *how much to eat* (and everything else).

You breast- or formula-feed smoothly, going by information coming from her about when, how often, how fast, and how much.

The division of responsibility for older babies

- You are still responsible for *what* you feed your child. You are *becoming* responsible for *when* and *where* to feed your child.
- Your child is *still and always* responsible for *how much* and *whether to* eat the foods you offer her.

Introducing solid food begins the transition from the infant's demand feeding to the child's meals-plus-snacks routine.

The division of responsibility for almost-toddlers

- You are responsible for *what*, *when*, and *where*.
- Your child is responsible for *how much* and *whether*.

Your child wants to feed herself soft pieces of mealtime food. Offer sit-down snacks to let her be hungry but not starved at mealtime.

The division of responsibility for toddlers

- You are responsible for *what*, *when*, and *where* to feed your child.
- Your child is responsible for how much and whether to eat the foods you put before her.

Your child wants to be her own little person, with eating as with everything else.

THE DIVISION OF RESPONSIBILITY IN FEEDING
for toddlers through adolescents

- You are responsible for *what*, *when*, and *where* to feed your child.
- Your child is responsible for *how much* and *whether* to eat of the foods you put before he.

Do your feeding jobs:	Trust your child to do her eating jobs:
• Choose and serve the food. • Provide regular meals and snacks. • Make eating times pleasant. • Show your child how to behave at meals. • Maintain structure. Offer your child water between regular meal- and snack-times but not other drinks or food. • Let your child grow in her way.	• She will eat. • She will eat the amount she needs. • She will learn to eat the food you eat. • She will learn to behave well at family meals. • She will grow up to have the body that is right for her.

Do your jobs with *feeding*, and trust your child to do her jobs with *eating*.

Trust your child to grow in the best way

Your child has a natural way of growing that is right for her. Her natural growth is in balance with her eating and moving. Maintain the division of responsibility in feeding and in activity *(next page)*. Trust her to do her part with eating, moving, and growing.

Your child's body shape and size are mostly inherited. Her height and weight are normal for her as long as she grows consistently, even if her growth plots at the extreme upper or lower ends of the growth charts. If her weight or height *abruptly* shifts up or down on her growth chart, it can mean a problem. Consult a health professional who understands the feeding relationship to rule out feeding, health, or parenting problems.

You won't know how your child's body will turn out until she is toward the end of her teen years. Trying to control or change it will likely create the very outcome you are trying to avoid! As long as you keep your nerve and maintain the division of responsibility with feeding and with activity, her growth may surprise you. The fat baby is likely to slim down. The small, ill, or growth-delayed child is likely to continue to do catchup growth well into her teen years and has a good chance of being bigger than you may expect.

The division of responsibility applies to the child who was prematurely born, is ill, or has special needs. Sections and stories throughout this booklet address those children.

Parent in the best way with physical activity

Children are born loving their bodies. They are curious about their physical capabilities and inclined to be active in a way that is right for them. Good parenting with activity preserves those qualities. Parents provide *structure*, *safety*, and *opportunities*. Children choose *how much* and *whether* to move and the *manner* of moving.

The division of responsibility in activity for infants

Provide your baby with a variety of positions, clothing, sights, and sounds. Then remain present and let your baby move.

- You are responsible for safe opportunities.
- Your baby is responsible for moving.

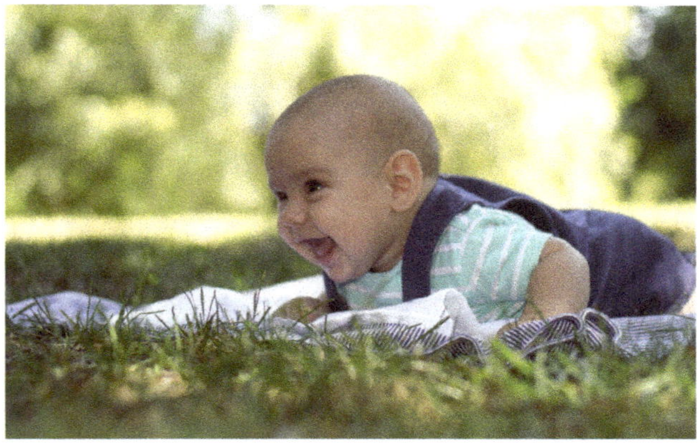

The division of responsibility in activity for older babies

Your child has built into him the drive to roll over, sit, stand, crawl, and walk. He will do it all when he is ready.

- You are responsible for keeping him safe.
- Your child is responsible for getting ready to move and for moving.

THE DIVISION OF RESPONSIBILITY IN ACTIVITY
for toddlers

- You are responsible for *structure, safety,* and *opportunities.*
- Your child is responsible for *how, how much,* and *whether* she moves.

Do your jobs:	Trust your child to do his jobs:
• Develop your tolerance for commotion—and your judgment about how much is too much. • Provide safe places for activity your child enjoys. • Have fun and rewarding family activities. • Set limits on TV and computer-like media but not on books, artwork, or other quiet activities. • Don't let your child watch media in her room.	• Your child will be active • She will be active in a way that is right for her.

Feeding stories: the first 2 years

Parents who follow the division of responsibility swear by it. Those who are new to it wonder whether it can possibly be right. Here is what parents say about the division of responsibility in feeding.

The division of responsibility pays off

We have been following the division of responsibility since both our children were born. Recently, we have been eating out more because we have been traveling. Because Henry, age 3, and Clara, age 1, sit with us at dinner each night and eat what we eat, they have been so good in restaurants. For my birthday we went to a nice restaurant, and they did so well it was actually fun. I was so proud of them, and the waiters were impressed!

Trust your child to grow

Josh was born 2 months prematurely. After we got him home, we followed his lead with his sleeping and eating. It was hard and scary, but during his first 2 months his weight gradually went up toward the third percentile. We felt like such failures when his doctor said he should grow faster! We tried to feed Josh more and more often. We even tried to wake him up to eat, which was almost impossible. After a miserable 4 months, Josh's weight was worse! So, we went back to trusting him, and he went back to gaining weight. Our doctor had kept Josh alive, so we felt bad ignoring her orders. Believing in Josh must have been hard and scary for her, as well.

Some children are big, and that is okay

When my daughter weighed almost 10 pounds at birth, I thought she would be fat when she grew up. I tried not to let her eat too much, even though she was fussy and hard to settle down. She stayed just as big, and by the time she became a toddler, she begged for food all day long. Then I learned about the division of responsibility and that not letting her eat as much as she wanted made her afraid of going hungry. At first it was scary to let her eat so much, but then her eating settled down. Now she is slimming down. That is fine, but the bottom line is that I like her body just the way it is, and I trust her to grow her way.

Children with special needs can be trusted

Bobby's newborn blood tests showed he had cystic fibrosis (CF). After he started taking digestive enzymes, his growth climbed to about the thirtieth weight percentile and stayed there. But the CF clinic stressed getting him to the fiftieth percentile, so I tried to feed him more. The more I pressured, the less he ate until he refused his bottle altogether and his weight plummeted. When I heard about the division of responsibility, I thought, "What kind of crazy person would come up with that? Bobby must eat!" But it had helped other parents and children, so I gathered my courage and did it. Within 3 days he began eating again, feeding went back to being a joy, and his growth went back up to the thirtieth percentile. I think the worst was losing my trust in Bobby to do his part with eating. Although Bobby has a "serious" form of CF, he is amazingly healthy.

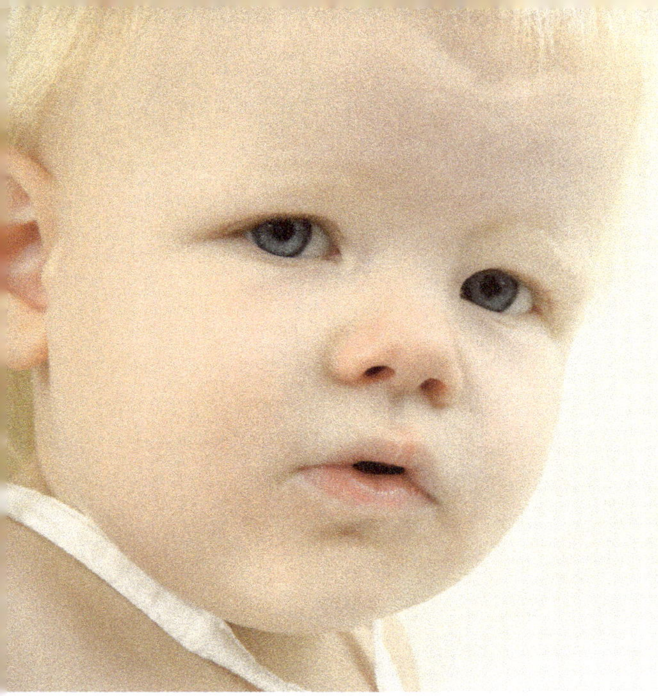

3

Cultivate your curiosity.
Get to know your child.

3. Understand your child's development and temperament

Knowing your child's developmental tasks at different stages will help you to understand your child and parent in the best way.

- **Homeostasis:** As a newborn, he learns to be calm and alert. You learn to respect his capabilities, to set aside your agenda, and to follow his lead.
- **Attachment:** After the first few months, he learns to love and to bond with you. You feel your love for him and show it by paying attention to him and doing what he wants.
- **Separation-individuation:** Toward the middle of the first year and into the second and third years, he learns that he is his own little person, separate from you. You provide structure and limits and then let him do it himself.

The first 8–12 weeks: Homeostasis

Doing what your baby wants you to do helps him be calm and alert so he can eat well. He shows signs that tell you when he needs to wake up, to sleep, to eat, and to stop eating. Watch for those signs, and do what he needs. You will not spoil him. You cannot spoil a tiny baby.

2–6 months: Attachment

Show your baby you love him by feeding when and how he wants to eat. He still needs help being calm and alert, but now he is learning to love. You and he take turns talking and smiling. You wait while he takes a breather and gets ready to talk more. Again, do not worry about spoiling him. You cannot spoil a little baby.

All the developmental tasks work together

Like a jazz band, one task takes center stage as the others "play" in the background. Feeding your newborn on demand lets him get started on separation-individuation by experiencing himself as a separate person. Following the division of responsibility in feeding lets your toddler continue to work on homeostasis. It takes some children longer than others to calm down!

5–9 months: Separation-individuation

Your older baby is interested in *things*, and he wants to see what is going on around him. This is the start of separation-individuation. He loves you as much as ever and wants you near, but it is not just the two of you anymore. He will suddenly sit up and look around in the middle of a nipple-feeding. He drains a bottle or breast in a hurry—he has things to do! Your introducing him to solid food goes right along with his interest in *things*.

7–15 months: Separation-individuation

Your almost-toddler cares deeply about *doing it herself*. One day, she will suddenly refuse the spoon, grab at it, and refuse foods she has enjoyed before. She will be happiest—and you will too—if you let her feed herself. Let her use her fingers as best she can. Do not try to feed her, or she will fuss and not eat. She is not being naughty. She still loves you and needs you. She still enjoys the food. In fact, if you let her feed herself, she will eat almost anything.

11–24 months: Separation-individuation

Your toddler learns to be part of the family at the same time as he can still be his own little person. Instead of dropping everything to feed him as you did when he was a baby, establish structure. He can learn to wait a bit to eat so he can join in with family meals. But don't let him wait too long or get too hungry. Give him sit-down snacks between meals. Since he will likely change suddenly from being a *happy-to-eat-anything* almost-toddler to a *picky* toddler, you may think there is something wrong. There isn't. He is just being a toddler.

Don't forget to have fun

Enjoy your child, cultivate your curiosity, and take pleasure from watching him grow up. Do not get caught in an agenda for what or how your child will eat or how he will grow, or it will spoil your fun. Do your jobs, then relax. Trust your child to do his part with eating, moving, and growing.

If your child was prematurely born

It is harder for a premature baby to become and stay calm and alert. What happened in the hospital was upsetting for her. On top of that, her nervous system is still not quite mature. It takes time, but you can get on her wavelength with feeding.

Her developmental stages will come along later and more slowly. She will master her sleeping and waking, learn to love, and insist on being her own little person the same as any other child. She will just take longer to move through the stages.

If your child was (is) ill or has special needs

The advice in this booklet applies to you and your child. You can still trust your child to learn and grow. Her developmental stages may come along later and she may master each stage more slowly, but they *will* come along and she *will* master them. You may be told that she can't regulate her food intake and won't grow up with eating like other children, but that is simply not true. You can trust her and follow a division of responsibility in feeding her. At the same time as you must be attentive to medical, developmental, and oral-motor issues, your feeding challenges will mostly come about because your child is a *child*, not because she has special needs.

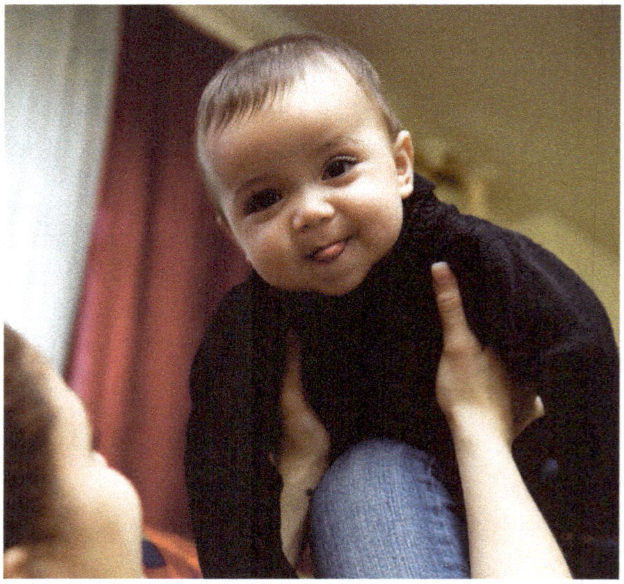

Your baby's temperament

Your baby was born with a certain temperament. You do not cause him to be that way. Get to know him and let yourself love him just the way he is. Understanding his temperament helps you be more patient with him—and with yourself! Keep in mind that he will not always be that way! If you do a good job with feeding, your slow-to-warm-up baby will become more flexible, and your uptight baby will become easier to please.

If your child is:	Here is what you can do to help:
Easy-going: Relaxed, calm, and easy to please with clear signs. Eats and sleeps regularly.	Go by your baby's signs. Know that you can trust him to show you what to do for him.
Slow-to-warm-up: Takes a while to get used to new things. Might not act pleased or happy, even when you get it right.	Do what *most* babies like, even if it does not seem to work. Offer lots of chances to learn to like new things. Don't get pushy. Stop when he shows signs that he wants to stop, but keep offering chances to learn.
Uptight: Wound up, touchy, and hard to figure out. His signs are not clear, except for being upset, and anything new upsets him! You cannot know ahead of time when he will eat or sleep, be fussy or happy.	Do what *most* babies like, even if it does not work at first. Keep trying, but know that his getting upset is not your fault or his. Know that he probably will not do the same thing twice. Be as calm and steady as you can. Get help if you need it.

The "difficult" baby

The "difficult" baby is uptight in the extreme. He cries a lot, cries loudly, is very difficult to soothe, and has trouble falling asleep, staying asleep, and waking up enough to eat well. First, some encouragement: "Difficult" babies who are parented well during the early months and years show the least behavior problems and greatest social skills of all children as first graders. In the meantime, if it *seems* hard, it is because it *is* hard. "Difficult" babies have a lot of trouble establishing homeostasis, trouble that persists for at least the first year and probably longer. Reread what it says on page 7 about *homeostasis* and about the *newborn*. Study the next chapter, *How to feed your newborn and infant*, and do the very best job of feeding you possibly can. Study your child's sleep states and hunger cues and follow them as best you can. Concentrate on the *quality* of feeding, not the *quantity* of food. You will be an advice magnet, so be skeptical of all input, except "I can take him for a few hours." You will be told to stop breastfeeding (or scolded for *not* breastfeeding), encouraged to keep trying formulas or nipples until you find one that "works," advised to put him on a schedule, or told to feed certain amounts. All of these strategies undermine his homeostasis and make the problem worse, not better.

Feeding and parenting your toddler

Your child loves you and wants to grow up to be just like you. He wants to learn to eat the food you eat. He will do best when you give him both love and limits—you do your jobs with feeding and let him do his jobs with eating.

What your child wants and needs:	What to do as a parent:
He wants to do well with eating.	Plan meals with both familiar and unfamiliar food. Let him eat or not eat from what you offer.
He needs pleasant mealtimes.	Talk about something else besides food. Help him learn to make conversation. Don't scold.
He needs to feel independent.	Help him get served, then don't interfere. Don't wipe, tidy, arrange, encourage, remind, suggest, or insist.
He wants to eat like you do.	Provide him with the same place setting you use—child-sized if you can. Let him learn by watching how you manage your silverware and napkin. Don't pester him—he is doing his best.
He wants to do it himself.	Let him serve himself. Teach him to dish up a little at a time, put the serving spoon back in the bowl, and pass the bowl to the next person. Keep extra spoons handy—learning takes a while!
He needs to know you approve.	Recognize when he does well. But don't make a big deal about it or he will think, "I must be stupid."
He will test the rules.	His behavior is negative if it interferes with your having a pleasant meal. Matter-of-factly tell him to stop. Excuse him from the meal if he persists.

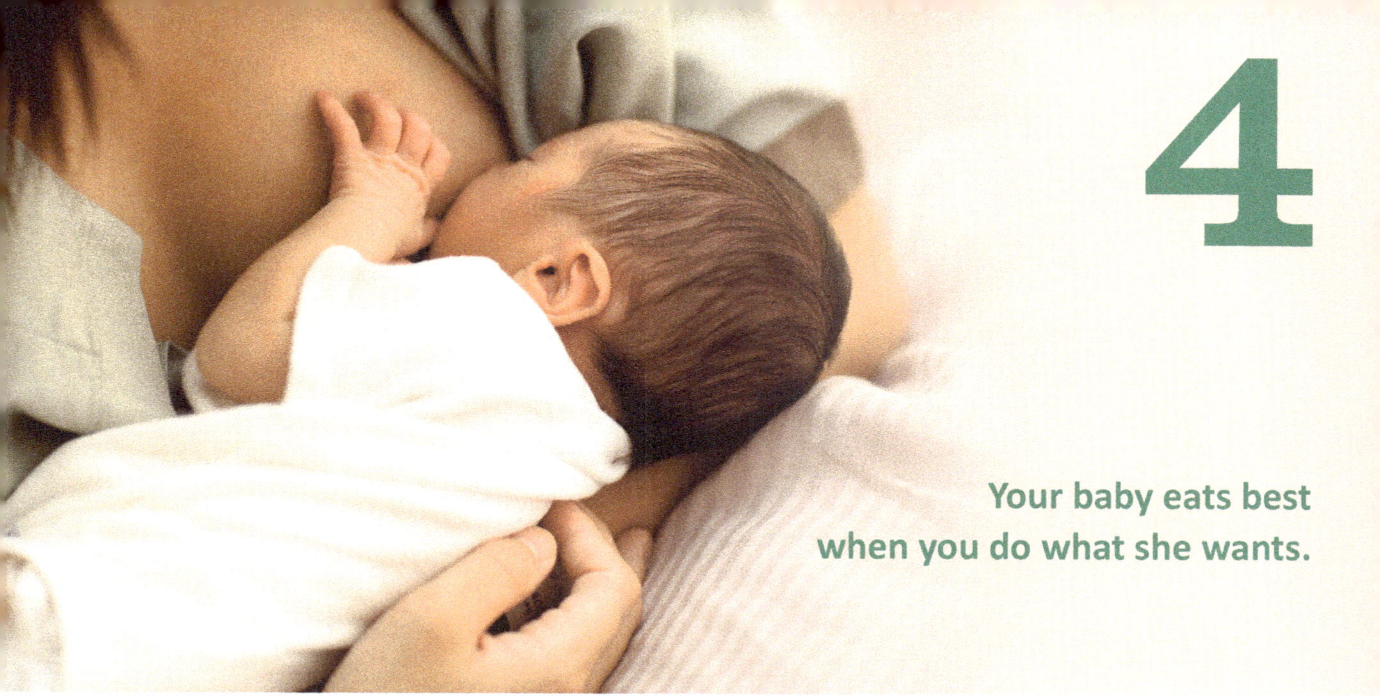
4
Your baby eats best
when you do what she wants.

4. How to feed your newborn and infant

Feed based on *what your baby can do*, not how old she is. Go at your baby's rate. Enjoy cuddling and nipple-feeding. Start solids at the right time: not too early, not too late. Some babies are ready early for mushy, semisolid foods from the spoon. Other babies are months older before they get ready.

During her first year to 18 months, your child moves through 2 phases in feeding:

- The *nipple only* phase for newborns and infants, usually up to about 6 months old.
- The *transition to family meals* phase for older babies and almost-toddlers.

Do not put cereal in the bottle. If your baby cannot eat from the spoon, she is not ready for solid foods and does not need the cereal.

When your child:	She is ready for:
• Cuddles • Roots for the nipple • Sucks	Nipple-feeding from the breast or bottle
• Sits up—alone or with support • Opens her mouth for the spoon • Closes her lips over the spoon • Keeps most of the food in her mouth • Swallows	Nipple-feeding from the breast or bottle *and* Mushy food that you feed her from the spoon

Does your baby need to eat, sleep, or talk?

Your baby eats and sleeps best if you do what she wants. Let her sleep until she is ready to get up. Help her wake up to get ready to eat. Feed her right away when she is ready. Help her stay awake through the whole feeding by looking at her, talking quietly to her, and stroking her in a way she likes. Put her to bed when she is sleepy and ready for a nap.

Your baby's sleeping and waking:	Here is what to do:
In ***quiet sleep***, she lies still and breathes deeply and evenly.	Let her sleep. She is sleeping deeply and will sleep for a while.
In ***active sleep***, she moves around, makes sounds, breathes fast or slowly.	Wait to see what happens. She might wake up, or she might go back to quiet sleep again.
Drowsy after sleeping, her eyes are open, but she looks sleepy. She fusses a little.	Wait a bit. If she keeps her eyes open or keeps fussing, get her up. Help her wake up. Hold her. Change her diaper. Talk with her.
Wide awake and calm, her eyes are wide open, she looks bright, and she is relaxed.	Feed her. She will eat best when she is awake and calm.
Drowsy after eating and playing, she looks sleepy and is relaxed.	Put her to bed and let her put herself to sleep. She may fuss a little, but not much.
Upset and crying, she is stiff and looks unhappy.	Comfort her. Help her calm down. Feed her if she wants to eat. She may need to fuss herself to sleep.

What sleep cycles look like

Sometimes Kari sleeps quietly, but most of the time she snorts and sniffs and thrashes about. I used to jump with every sound, and when she was quiet, I kept checking to be sure she was still breathing! At first, I picked her up as soon as she cried, but she was too sleepy to eat well or she got really fussy. It turns out she was in active sleep and I was interrupting her sleep cycle. When she is ready to wake up, her eyes stay open, and she has a certain kind of cry. She quiets right down when I pick her up and by the time I change her diaper, she is wide awake and ready to eat. She eats well and doesn't get fussy. Afterwards, she stays awake a while, and when she gets drowsy, I put her down and she puts herself to sleep. She fusses a bit, but it seems more like she is singing herself to sleep than really crying.

Feed so your baby can eat well

Your baby eats best and feels best about you—and about eating—when you pay attention to her and do what she wants. Guide feeding by paying attention to her signs of hunger and fullness. Newborns usually eat every 2 hours, but keep the timing right for your baby by making each feeding as good as can be. Read her sleep and awake signs. Help her stay calm and awake while she eats.

What to do at the *start* of a feeding

- ***Feed when she wants to eat and is wide awake and calm.***
  Don't try to feed her on a schedule or when you think of it. Don't feed when she is drowsy or upset.
- ***Ask her to open her mouth by touching her cheek or lips or showing her the nipple.***
  Don't pry open her mouth. Don't plop in the nipple when she yawns, laughs, or cries.

What to do *during* a feeding

- ***Keep her head, back, and shoulders in a straight line; keep the bottle nipple filled.***
  Don't let her body twist or droop. Don't let her suck an empty nipple. Don't prop the bottle.
- ***Sit still; keep the feeding smooth and steady.***
  Don't jiggle her or jiggle the breast or bottle. Don't stop feeding to wipe, burp, or play.
  When she needs burping, she stops eating and looks uncomfortable.
- ***Let her eat her way—fast or slowly, steady, or start-and-stop.***
  Don't make her hurry up or slow down.
- ***Talk to her or touch her in a way that she likes and that helps her to stay awake.***
  Don't talk loudly or in an unpleasant voice. Don't jiggle or tickle.

What to do at the *end* of a feeding

- ***Let her eat a lot or a little.*** Don't make her eat a certain amount.
- ***Let her rest for a bit and then offer the nipple again to see whether she wants to eat more.***
  Don't assume she is full if she stops and looks around. She may want to look at you or rest.
- ***Work toward having her be awake at the end of the feeding.***
  Don't deliberately feed her to sleep.

What to do *after* a feeding

- ***Talk or play a while; keep her close while you eat or go about your day; put her to bed when she is calm and drowsy and let her put herself to sleep.***
  Don't wait until she is upset and fussy to put her down. Don't routinely rock, walk, or feed her to sleep.

If your baby was born prematurely, is ill, or has special needs

Because of hospital procedures that were done to her mouth, your baby is likely to be touchy about eating. It also will be hard to read her signs. Her prematurity or special needs may make her seem slow to warm up or even uptight. You can get on her wavelength, but it takes time. Even though she is tiny or ill, she can show you when she is hungry and when she is full.

It is hard for your baby to wake up. Once she is awake, it is hard for her to become calm and alert. Once she is calm and alert, it is easy for her to slip into being upset. You will be able to help her with all of this, but it is challenging.

Helping your baby do a good job with eating:

- ***Use nipples and formula the same way all the time.***
  If she is still in the hospital, try to see that she gets a chance to nipple-feed or at least to suck on a pacifier. If she is tube-fed, hold her and let her suck on a nipple at the same time. Settle on one type of nipple, and then use it all the time. Use the formula your health worker recommends. Unless you *have* to, don't switch from one formula to another.

- ***Don't follow a schedule or try to get your baby to eat a certain amount.***
  Concentrate on the *quality* of feeding rather than the *quantity* she eats. Your baby will eat best when you make each feeding as good as it can be. Study her sleeping and waking to learn her special cues. Be especially quiet, slow, and low-key with her. Do your best to follow her feeding cues.

- ***Look for your baby's hard-to-understand feeding signals.***
  She may show she is hungry (or full) by losing interest in talking and playing, getting fussy, becoming stiff or arching her back, or going to sleep. Follow her signs as best you can. Think about what happened before and between feedings to help figure out what her signs mean. Over time, her signs will become more readable, and you will get good at reading them.

- ***Let her be in control.***
  Wait to feed until she is quiet and alert and shows you she is hungry. Touch her cheek or show her the nipple and wait for her to open her mouth. Stop feeding when she shows you she is full.

- ***Don't be in a hurry to start solids.***
  It may be weeks before nipple-feeding goes smoothly. Take time to enjoy it before you move on to the next step. *Offer solids based on what your baby can do, not how old she is* (page 11).

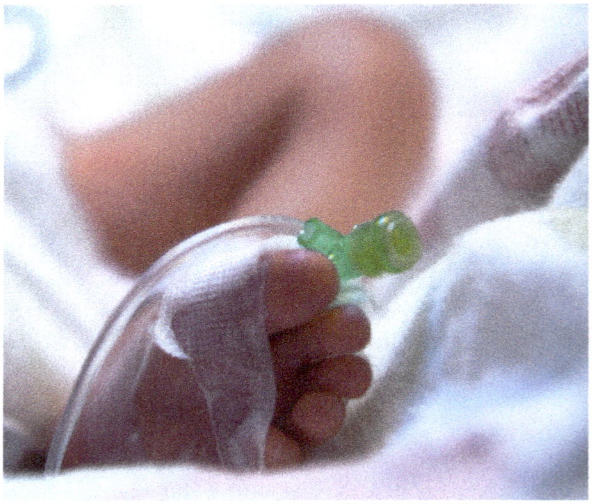

Feeding stories: the newborn or infant

Every baby is different. Let your baby eat how he wants.

A baby who knew how (and one who didn't)

Sena was born knowing how to nurse, and her mother thought she had the touch! Sena was settled and relaxed, she had a good suck, and there was plenty of breastmilk. She slept well and woke up every three or four hours to eat again. But Sena's little brother Tommy was a whole different story! He never did the same thing twice, needed help learning how to latch on and to suck, and had trouble sleeping and waking up. Even though she was experienced, his mother still had a lot of learning to do.

The hungry baby

Lucy's mother thought her baby was done eating when she finished her bottle. But Lucy would fuss and be unhappy at the end of feedings. When her mother learned of the division of responsibility, she realized that Lucy was still hungry. She made Lucy another bottle so she could eat as much as she wanted. Lucy grew better and was happier—and so was her mother!

Big babies know how to eat and grow

Joseph's mother was told to restrict her chubby, fast-growing, 3-month-old baby to 5 rather than his usual 7 or 8 breastfeedings a day. So she postponed feeding until Joseph got so upset that she *had* to give in and feed him. But her breastmilk started drying up and they were both unhappy, so she went back to feeding him on demand. Feeding went back to being great, but she worried a lot that not following doctor's orders would make Joseph fat. She was glad she had followed her own instincts when she learned that not giving her baby enough to eat was likely to make him fatter rather than thinner.

Tiny babies know how to eat and grow

Margene was born 3 weeks early, and her weight plotted below the third percentile. She ate every 2 or 3 hours, had lots of wet diapers, and had 5 or 6 poops a day. But her doctor said she was *failing to thrive*, (a serious diagnosis that means a child is eating and growing poorly) and told her mother to give her formula after every breastfeeding. After that, breastfeeding didn't go so well. Margene grew, but she didn't do any catchup growing, and feeding was such a worry and hassle! Margene's parents were upset when they found out that all the hassle probably made Margene eat and grow less well, not better. But they were glad to know they could go back to trusting Margene to eat and grow. They guessed that tiny babies scare everyone, even doctors with lots of experience, and scared people tend to put pressure on feeding.

Start now with family meals

Even a newborn can join in with family meals when you prop her up safely nearby or hold her while you eat. *Have family-friendly meals* (page 24), starting right now. Within months, your baby will be ready to join you!

Breastfeeding and formula-feeding

When you follow the division of responsibility, babies get their nutritional and emotional needs met with both breastfeeding and formula-feeding. With both, babies grow up to be healthy, intelligent, and thin, fat, or in between. To do a good job with either breastfeeding or formula-feeding, be comfortable with your feeding method. Don't let anybody else decide for you. You know yourself and your baby best, and you can rely on your own judgment. To help you decide, learn about breastfeeding. Talk with someone who has breastfed. Try breastfeeding at first. Get help if you need it. If you like it (or it is even just okay) and if your breastfeeding partnership with your baby works, breastfeed. If you don't like it and/or it doesn't work, you don't have to breastfeed.

How to breastfeed

Breastfeeding takes some learning. Here is what you need to know:

- Your baby can nurse right away, and gets the colostrum your breasts make at first.
- Your breastmilk comes in when your baby is 2 to 5 days old. At first there may be too much, but soon you will make only as much as your baby empties from your breasts.
- Your breast makes the milk higher up and "lets down" the milk into the nipple. Your breasts may or may not tingle when your milk lets down.
- You will know your baby is getting milk. You can see and hear her swallow, and you can see her pees and poops. Look for six to eight wet diapers a day and many poopy ones.
- You will know whether your baby is not eating enough. There will not be enough pees and poops, and she will not gain weight. Concentrate on making each feeding better, not on getting more into her. Read her sleep and awake signs. Talk with her in a voice she likes to help her stay awake, calm, and alert while she eats.
- There will be some hungry days when your baby nurses more and your breastmilk supply catches up.

Feed yourself so you can breastfeed your baby

- Have regular meals with food you enjoy. You need energy to make breastmilk and to take care of your baby and yourself.
- Keep drinks with caffeine down to one or two a day. More can make your baby jittery.
- Keep alcohol down to one drink a day. Wait 2 hours before you breastfeed.
- If your baby gets stomachaches easily, try cutting out cabbage, cauliflower, broccoli, or collard greens. You might also have to stay away from cooked dried beans.

Vitamin D and fluoride

- Talk with your health care provider about whether your baby needs supplements of fluoride or vitamin D.

Hungry days

Your baby will have hungry days as she grows and needs more breastmilk. Some babies have one hungry day a week. Some have two hungry days every several weeks. Some seem hungry all the time! Hungry days can be tough, tiring days. Even if you don't have much milk, your baby's sucking more tells your breasts to make more milk. Let her eat every hour or two—or more often—even if she does not get much. After a day or two, your breasts will make more milk. Pumping breastmilk and feeding it from a bottle doesn't stimulate breasts any more or give your baby any more milk.

How to feed from the bottle

Whether you put formula or breastmilk in the bottle, bottle-feeding takes some learning. Here is what you need to know:

- ***Be consistent:*** Your baby knows the world through her mouth. She gets attached to the taste, feel, and temperature of her feedings. Change upsets her.
- ***Use standard baby formula***: You can buy it in the grocery store, drug store, or discount store. Measure and mix just as it says on the label. Don't measure in bottles with plastic liners.
- ***Use easy-to-clean bottles:*** Avoid fancy shapes. Use glass bottles, or use plastic bottles or liners made with nontoxic materials.
- ***Use one type of nipple and check that it works right:*** Pick one nipple shape and use it all the time. Turn the bottle upside down to see that drops come out one right after the other but not in a steady stream.

Remember how important you are

Every baby is born with the longing to be understood, and out of your understanding grows love. You show your baby you love and understand her when you pay attention and feed based on what she wants and needs. Follow your baby's sleep cycles to time feeding. Base your feeding method—nipple, solids, or finger-feeding—based on what your baby can *do*, not how old she is. Follow the division of responsibility, faithfully doing your jobs with feeding and trusting your child to do her part with eating. Problem-solve based on the division of responsibility and a clear understanding of normal child eating behavior. Avoid rules about when and what to feed: Rules make you ignore your baby and doubt your judgment.

- ***Keep nipples and bottles clean:*** Scrub in hot soapy water and rinse them well. For the first month, boil nipples, bottles, and the water used for mixing formula for 3 minutes.
- ***Make sure the water is safe:*** Have home wells tested.
- ***Refrigerate formula after you open it:*** This applies to powdered as well as liquid formula. Throw away any formula left in the bottle after a feeding.
- ***Change gradually:*** If you have to change formulas or change from breastmilk to formula, do it gradually. For a day or two, mix 1 ounce of the new with 6 to 8 ounces of the old. Then for a day or two, use 2 ounces of the new, and so on, until you have made the change.
- ***Have regular meals with food you enjoy:*** You need energy to take care of your baby and yourself.
- ***Fluoride:*** Talk with your health care provider about whether your baby needs a fluoride supplement.

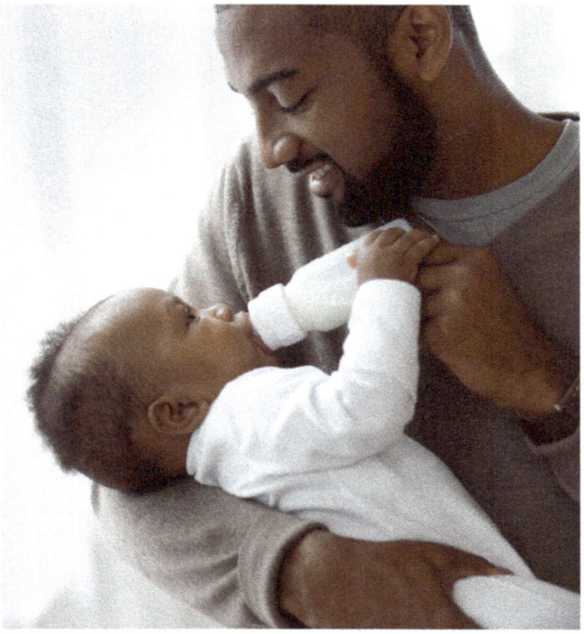

Your baby eats best when you do what she wants.

Teaching your breastfed baby to take a bottle

Even if you prefer to breastfeed only, you may sometimes need to use a bottle. By the time she is 4 to 6 weeks old, your baby will be so good at breastfeeding that teaching her to suck from a bottle will not confuse her. She will learn to switch easily between breast and bottle. But she does need time to get used to the idea. Here is how to help her:

- ***Get ready:*** Put a small amount of pumped breastmilk* or formula in the bottle. Have your baby be a little hungry but not so hungry she is desperate to eat. Have someone besides Mom offer the bottle so your baby does not expect to breastfeed.
- ***Be patient:*** Plan on at least 10 practice sessions before your baby takes even a few swallows. She has a lot to learn. The rubber nipple does not feel like a breast nipple. To work the rubber nipple, she has to suck and swallow in a whole different way. If there is formula in the bottle, it tastes different from breastmilk. Don't get pushy or it will slow her learning.
- ***Be consistent:*** Pick out one type of nipple, formula, and bottle and use them all the time. Don't switch around. Each switch requires more learning.
- ***Introduce the new nipple:*** Touch the nipple to her cheek or lip and let her open her mouth. After she opens her mouth, squeeze a drop on the nipple. Place the nipple gently in her mouth and let her decide what to do with it.
- ***Do what she wants:*** She might or might not open her mouth for the nipple, and she might or might not try to suck. Stop right away when she shows you she wants to stop.
- ***Understand how she learns:*** She will not do, not do, not do, and then she will do. Don't get pushy. Just keep giving her chances to learn.

*For more information about storing breastmilk, check out the breastfeeding chapter in ***Child of Mine: Feeding with Love and Good Sense.***

To heat or not to heat?

Either warm or cold is fine, but do it the same way every time. To heat it, put the bottle of formula in a pan of hot water or hold it under hot running water. *Microwaving is not recommended.* If you do it, be extra careful. Microwaving causes hot spots that could burn your baby:

- Leave the nipple or cap *off* the bottle during microwaving.
- Heat 4-ounce bottles no more than 30 seconds, and heat 8-ounce bottles no more than 45 seconds.
- Put the nipple on and turn the bottle upside down 10 times to mix the hot and cold spots.

Whichever method you use to heat the formula, test the temperature by putting a few drops on the inside of your wrist. If it is the right temperature, you will not be able to feel it. If it feels hot, it is *too* hot.

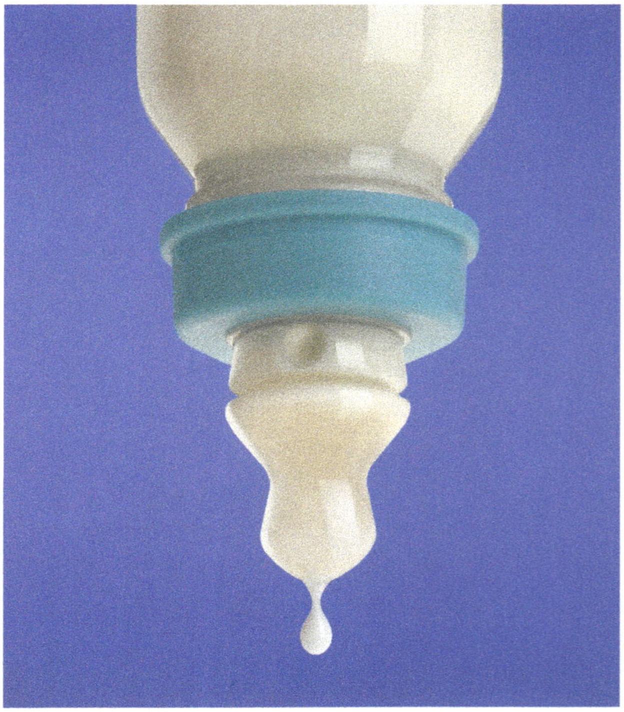

Drops should follow closely, but not be a steady stream.

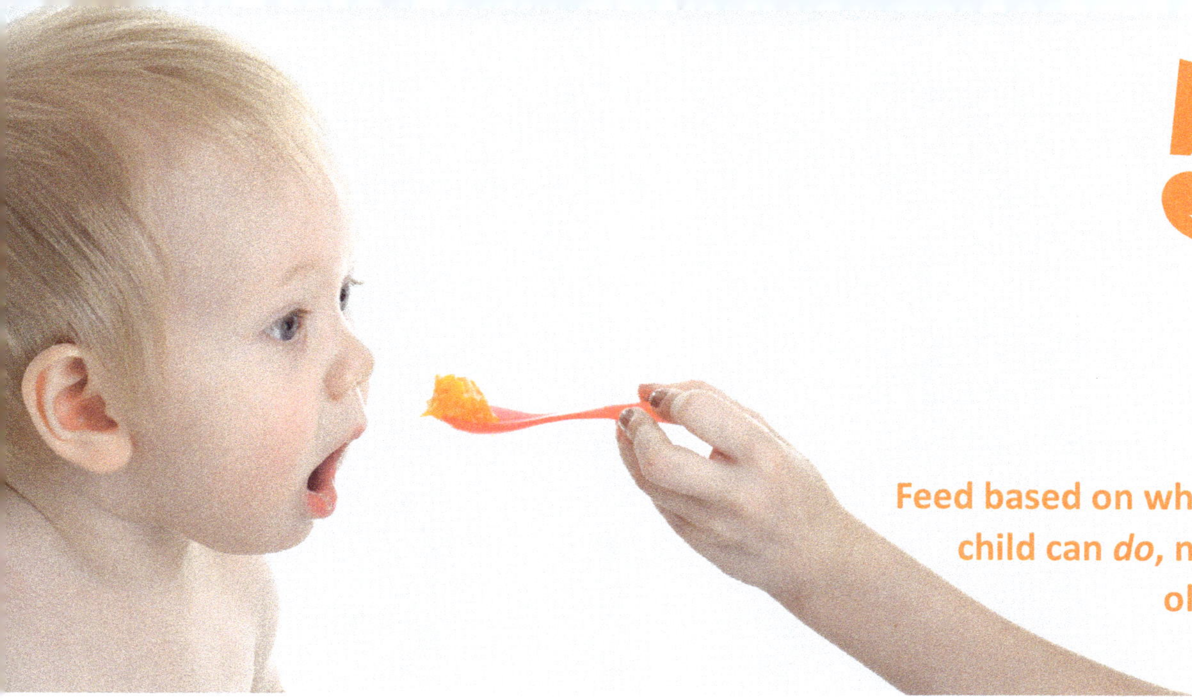

5

Feed based on what your child can *do*, not how old he is.

5. How to feed your older baby and toddler

Make the transition to family meals.

Once you start solid food, what and how you feed your child continuously changes until he finger-feeds himself and joins in with family meals. You build on his increased regularity with eating to move away from the demand feeding of infancy to the meals-plus-snacks routine of the older child.

Offer solids based on what your baby can *do*, not how old he is.

Ignore rules about when to start and progress solids and what to feed. Rules about feeding make you ignore your baby and doubt your own judgment. Many babies show the signs of readiness to start solid foods by 5 or 6 months, move quickly through thicker, lumpier food and finger food, and have the finger and mouth skills to feed themselves step 4 family food at family meals by age 7 to 10 months. Others may start at about the usual time but take it more slowly and get to step 4 when they are in their second or even third year. Still others can't be bothered with spoon-feeding and wait to eat solid foods until they can finger-feed themselves family food.

Cultivate your curiosity.

How will your baby move through this process? Will he *love* spoon-feeding, like Jonathan, or not want to be bothered, like Sebastian? *See Feeding stories: starting solid foods* (page 22). Or will he be somewhere in between? However he reacts to his first solid food is right, so relax and enjoy it.

When your child:	He is ready for:
• Cuddles • Roots for the nipple • Sucks	Nipple-feeding from the breast or bottle
• Sits up—alone or with support • Opens his mouth for the spoon • Closes his lips over the spoon • Keeps most of the food in his mouth • Swallows	Nipple-feeding from the breast or bottle *and* Mushy food that you feed him from the spoon
• Picks up food but cannot let go • Keeps food in his mouth instead of swallowing right away • Moves the food to his jaws • Munches the food	Breastmilk or formula from the nipple or cup *and* Step 2 food: Thicker, lumpier food that you feed from the spoon
• Closes his lips around the rim of the cup • Picks up food, puts it in his mouth • Bites off food • Chews • Gags some but does not choke (if he can breathe, he is gagging and not choking)	Breastmilk, formula, or juice that you give him from the cup *and* Step 3 food: Small pieces of soft finger food and foods he bites or breaks off with his gums
• Uses his fingers to pick up food • Can chew and swallow • Can join in with family meals	Whole pasteurized milk from the cup *and* Step 4 food: Easy-to-chew and easy-to-swallow grown-up food

Getting to grown-up food: steps 1 and 2

Easy does it! You are starting solid food not because your baby *has* to have it, but to support his oral-motor development. Step 1 food teaches him to use his mouth to get food from the spoon and swallow it. Step 2 food teaches him to use his tongue to push lumps between his jaws and mush them. Don't worry if he does not have teeth. He does just fine with his gums.

- ***Feed him when he is a little hungry, between breasts or after part of a bottle.***
  Don't let him be too hungry or he will get upset.
- ***Pick one mushy food to start with and stick with it for a while.***
  Don't surprise him with new food too often.
- ***Sit him up in a high chair with his head facing straight forward so he can swallow well; maybe prop him up with pillows.***
  Don't have him leaning back or lying down. Don't make him turn his head to see or to reach the spoon.
- ***Sit right in front of him; hold the spoon about a foot away from his mouth.***
  Don't hold the spoon so close it feels pushy or so far away he cannot see it well.
- ***Wait to see whether he opens his mouth; put food on his lip.***
  Don't pry his lips open with the spoon. Don't plop the food in before he is ready.
- ***Feed the way he wants to eat—a little or a lot, fast or slow.***
  Don't make him hurry up or slow down. Don't stop feeding before he shows he is done.
- ***Look at him; pay attention to him; talk to him kindly and quietly.***
  Don't talk a lot, play, sing, watch TV. On the other hand, don't just sit there.
- ***Let him feed himself if he wants, even if he grabs the spoon or smears food.***
  Don't worry if he does not get much in his mouth.
- ***Stop when he shows you he is done, even if he did not eat.***
  Don't try to get him to eat when he turns away, closes up, or fusses.

Don't panic about gagging, but avoid choking

Gagging is a normal part of learning to eat. A child gags when food slips to the back of his tongue before he is ready to swallow. Choking is dangerous. It closes off the windpipe so your child cannot breathe. Have your health-care provider teach you first aid for choking. Feed to avoid choking:

- Teach him step by step to eat solid food.
- Wait to give steps 3 and 4 food until his mouth is ready.
- Always have a grown-up with him when he eats. Don't leave older children in charge.
- Keep eating times calm and quiet. Have him sit down when he eats.
- Avoid round foods and hard foods that can plug up his windpipe. (See Step 3: *Finger food* page 31)
- Don't let him go to bed with a bottle, cup, or food.

Feeding stories: starting solid foods

Every child learns to eat differently. All of these children became good eaters, because their parents trusted that they knew what they were doing and that eventually they would get around to eating.

"Fast" learner Jonathan

After his first bite of cereal, Jonathan put up a tremendous fuss. He yelled and cried with his mouth full and between bites. After some trial and error, his mother figured out he was insisting on "more, faster."

Prematurely born Archie

Archie was nine months old before he showed signs of solids readiness. He scowled ferociously and gagged pitifully the first time he got a tiny bit of cereal in his mouth. His mother stopped with that tiny bit, and the next day he scowled and gagged less and took a bit more.

"I will do it myself" Clara

Clara enjoyed her cereal well enough but only if she was allowed to hold the spoon. She would suck it off, then surrender it and allow it to be refilled.

"Let me at it" India

At 5-and-a-half months, India ate happily from the spoon. At 7 months, she refused to open up for it. Her mother thickened her baby cereal and put it on the high-chair tray. India figured out how to lower her mouth to the edge of the tray and scoop cereal in with whatever was handy: her hand, her arm, a spoon.

"Don't bother me" Sebastian

Sebastian was not interested in eating from the spoon, although he would smear globs of baby cereal around on his high-chair tray. He got in his mouth only what he sucked off his fingers. Once he tried India's method, but it did not interest him.

"Let's skip this kid stuff" Jenny

Jenny never did get around to eating semisolid food, even though her parents tried all the methods. She took an interest only when she could gum and swallow pieces of soft foods the grown-ups were eating. In fact, pizza was her big breakthrough!

"I am too full to eat" Christopher

Ten-month-old Christopher was not interested in being at the table or eating solid food. He was overdosing on nipple-feeding—every two or three hours, when he got upset about something, and twice at night. His parents worked toward using nipple-feedings for scheduled snacks and waited to nipple-feed until after meals. After that, Christopher caught on to eating family meals, and he ate so much he wasn't interested in after-meal nipple feedings.

Getting to grown-up food: steps 3 and 4

Eating step 3 food (soft finger food) and step 4 food (easy-to-chew grown-up food) lets your child join in with family meals and eat what everyone else is eating. Step 3 is the introduction phase, where you try your child out on first one and then another food and watch to be sure it doesn't make him sick. You enter step 3 when, along with spoon-feeding, you put a few Cheerios and soft pieces of other food on his high-chair tray and let him try to pick them up and eat them. You are in step 4 when you realize he is eating the same soft food you eat and regularly joining you at family meals!

As your child eats more solid food, he will lose interest in the breast or bottle. Work toward the meals-plus-snacks routine by offering food every 2 to 3 hours, with 3 meals a day and snacks between times. Don't wait for teeth. He does just fine with his gums.

What to do at the *start* of a feeding

- ***Time snacks and nipple-feedings so he can be hungry but not starved at mealtimes; snacks can be nipple-feedings or "big-boy" snacks.*** Don't let him panhandle for breastfeedings or eat or drink on the run. Don't let him drink anything except water in between times.
- ***Have meals and snacks be your idea.*** Don't wait for him to say "I am hungry" before you offer meals and snacks.
- ***Keep making food you enjoy; sooner or later he will learn to eat most foods.*** Don't cook for him; cook for yourself. Don't ask him what he wants you to make; that is your job, and he is too little to know. Don't try in any way to make him eat—eating is his job.

What to do *during* a feeding

- ***Give him a tablespoon or two of each food; let him have more if he wants.*** Don't give him a lot or not enough. Don't make him eat one food before he can have another.
- ***Eat with him; enjoy your own meal or snack.*** Don't go off and leave him while he eats.
- ***Let him eat his way—much or little, fast or slowly, fingers or spoon.*** Don't hurry him up or slow him down. Don't make him eat more or less.
- ***Talk about something else besides the food and his eating.*** Don't praise or scold him about his eating.
- ***Be good company; talk and answer; be easy-going.*** Don't ignore him, but don't make him the center of attention either. Don't watch TV, text, or make phone calls. Don't fuss at him for spills.
- ***Teach him to behave so you can have a nice meal; excuse him when he is done.*** Don't put up with bad behavior or make him stay at the meal in hopes he will eat.

Baby-led weaning

The book, *Baby-Led Weaning*, urges skipping spoon-feeding of steps 1 and 2 foods and introducing solids when a baby can finger-feed herself sticks of soft food (teething biscuits or specially made food from recipes in the book). Know your baby. To do her oral-motor learning, she may need to mosey through the steps and be introduced gradually to tastes and textures. On the other hand, she might only take an interest in solid food when she is allowed to feed herself. Or she might be somewhere in between. However she does it, she *will* learn to eat family food, and she *will* join in with family meals.

Have family-friendly meals

Your almost-toddler or toddler needs structure with food the same as with everything else in his life. He also needs to have control. To provide structure, have family meals and sit-down snacks. To give him control, let him decide what and how much to eat at those times.

A family meal is when you all sit facing one another and share the same food. You do not need a table—a blanket on the floor will do—and the food does not have to be fancy. You can cook from scratch, defrost it in the microwave, have food delivered, or order at a fast-food restaurant.

Get started with family meals by changing the *how* first; think about the *what* later—lots later. Make meals your idea—don't just offer them when somebody else wants something to eat. Remember whose meal it is. Prepare food you enjoy, and know that sooner or later your child will eat almost everything you eat.

First, get the meal habit

- Eat what you are eating now. Just have it at regular meal- and snack-times.
- Round up the family to eat together.
- Let everyone decide what and how much to eat from what you provide for the meal.
- Make mealtimes pleasant. Talk and enjoy each other. Don't scold or fight.

After that, you might crave a little variety

- Add on foods; don't take them away.
- Include one or two foods that each person (generally) enjoys and can fill up on, such as bread.
- Include fat when you cook and at mealtime to make food taste good. Fat with food also keeps you from getting hungry right away.
- Let everyone—including you—pick and choose from what is in the meal and eat what tastes good.
- Don't try to please all the eaters with every food. Don't get pushy with feeding.

Then you might be ready to do some planning

- Include all the food groups: Meat or other protein; grains; fruit or vegetable or both; and milk. Also include fatty foods such as butter, salad dressing, or gravy.
- Because grains are easy to enjoy and good to fill up on, be particularly careful to include plenty of "bread" or whatever your family considers bread: sliced bread, tortillas, pita, Indian flat bread, Asian pancakes or wraps, cornbread, biscuits, crackers, rice, or pasta. Although potatoes and corn are vegetables, they can go on this list.
- Pair familiar food with unfamiliar, favorite with not-so-favorite.

For more about providing family-friendly meals, see *Secrets of Feeding a Healthy Family: How to Eat, How to Raise Good Eaters, How to Cook.*

Drinking and eating on the go: Sippy cups, food pouches, and snack traps

Keep your feeding goal in mind: Helping your child to *grow up to be a good eater* (page 1), *not* getting-food-into-your-child right *now*. It doesn't matter if the food in the pouch, on-the-go cup (or bottle), or snack gadget is nutritious or even *organic*. Your child won't learn to be a good eater, and in the long run, his nutrition will suffer. Like other children, your child is likely to *love* slurping and munching on the go. But if you let him, expect this: He will have trouble knowing how much he needs to eat and may eat too little and grow too slowly or eat too much and grow too fast. He will behave poorly at family meals because he isn't hungry and can't be bothered. He won't learn to eat the food you eat because *his* special food, delivered in *his* special way, is more to his liking.

Feeding stories: the almost-toddler

When you follow the division of responsibility, the way your child eats step 3 and step 4 foods (pages 31 and 32) is likely to be fun, messy, and quirky. Enjoy it!

Mary wanted to eat what her parents ate

Eight-month-old Mary watched her parents eat and moved her mouth while they chewed. She loved chasing Cheerios around on her high-chair tray and gummed strips of toast. She was ready for more, but her parents felt that their pizza, hamburgers, fries, and burritos were not good for her. They were surprised to learn that toddlers who eat family foods have better nutrition than those who eat baby foods. So, Mary's parents learned to cool down their pizza and cut it into bite-sized pieces, to cut strips of hamburger for her, and to give her French fries that were not too crisp. They cut up fried chicken, burritos, and barbeque. Since Mary was eating what her parents usually ate, it was easy for them to add soft fruits and cooked vegetables. Mary loved it all.

Tobin wanted to do it himself

Thirteen-month-old Tobin was born with cognitive limitations and skeletal malformations. He did fine on nipple-feeding, but feeding him solid foods was "an all-day job," and he gagged a lot. So, instead of feeding Tobin separately, his parents decided to include him in family meals. They brought him to the table, propped him up in his high chair, and put small pieces of food in front of him. Tobin's face brightened up, he zeroed in on the food, and he struggled to pick it up. He quickly developed the muscle control he needed to feed himself, chew, and swallow, and he stopped gagging.

Isaac loved butter

Isaac got the idea of eating family meals when he discovered butter. He licked it off his bread and ate it like cheese when he could get his hands on it. His parents learned that recently weaned children eat butter because they need the calories. So, they let him have pieces of butter, which he enjoyed thoroughly, and that enjoyment helped him learn to eat other foods, including fruits and vegetables. Then one day, he stopped eating butter. He didn't need that many calories any more.

Adele *loved* to eat

Fourteen-month-old Adele *loved* to eat! She was the first to come to the family table and the last one to leave. While she ate, she seemed filled with delight and even moaned softly! Adele's parents were amused by her eating, but they did not make an issue about it because they did not want to spoil it for her. They also loved her chubby little body. They could see that Adele was strong and active and that she knew what she was doing with her eating and growing.

Annie had known hunger

Annie, adopted from another country when she was 14 months old, ate like a starving person and ate a *lot*. Annie's parents understood that she had known hunger and desperately needed to be reassured that she would get enough to eat. They followed a division of responsibility, offered plenty of filling and enjoyable food at planned meals and snacks, let her eat as much as she wanted, and kept their nerve through her gobbling and occasional vomiting. When Annie begged for food between times, they reassured her, "it will soon be time to eat, and then you can have as much as you want." Annie recovered from her terror, began eating at a more moderate pace, and stopped throwing up.

The toddler's eating is quirky

The toddler's quirky eating puts a lot of pressure on parents to make errors in feeding. After loving to eat as an almost-toddler, the toddler suddenly becomes skeptical about new food (even if you know he has eaten it before), eats less (because he grows more slowly), and says "no" to food (often at the same time as he eats it). He refuses meals, begs for cookies right after, and then has a tantrum when you refuse. After the storm, he likes you better than ever. Hang in there! He will eat what the rest of the family eats, but it has to be *his* idea.

Toddlers eat what they need

Provided you maintain the structure of meals and snacks, over a week or two your toddler eats what he needs and eats enough to grow well. He can learn to eat new food. With your maintaining the division of responsibility in feeding (and a few showdowns), he behaves at mealtime so you enjoy having him there. Here is what a toddler's competent eating looks like:

- ***Erratic:*** At times, he will not eat much—a few tastes, swallows, finger fulls, or bites. Other times, he will eat more than you can imagine.
- ***Picky:*** He won't eat some of everything in the meal but only one or two foods.
- ***Fickle:*** What he eats one day, he ignores another.
- ***Cautious:*** If he has not seen it before (or *thinks* he has not), he probably will not eat it. But he sneaks up on it. He watches you eat it, looks at it, puts it in his mouth, and takes it out again.
- ***Messy:*** He drops food, smears it, gets it all over his face, and makes his place look like a disaster area.

Have family-friendly meals (page 24)

Eat with your child; don't just feed him. *Avoid pressure* (page 28). Your getting pushy will slow down his learning rather than speed it up.

Avoid common feeding mistakes

- **Limiting the menu to the food he accepts:** He is learning to eat the food *you* eat.
- **Playing games to get him to eat:** He will play games right back. You will do all sorts of embarrassing things—and he still will not eat.
- **Keeping him at the table when he shows he is done in hopes he will eat more:** He *won't* eat more, he *will* behave badly, and he *will* learn to dislike family meals.
- **Short-order cooking; asking him what he wants:** He does not know what he wants to eat until it is in front of him—and maybe not then.
- **Leaving out little dishes of food for him to grab when he walks by:** He needs to eat with the family.
- **Waiting to feed him until he tells you he is hungry:** He is too busy to know he is hungry until he falls apart or has a tantrum. Then he will be too upset to eat.
- **Using food to calm things down:** Instead, give attention, a hug, or a nap. Sticking to the meals-plus-snacks schedule helps you avoid feeding for emotional reasons.

Be considerate without catering

You can expect your child to come to the meal, but *you cannot make him eat*, even when the food is familiar. Just say (and *mean* it), "You don't have to eat. Just sit here and keep us company for a few minutes while *we* eat." Do make—and enforce—a rule about not eating or drinking anything (except for water) until snack-time.

Catering to your child's food whims does not do him any favors. Making special food or limiting the menu to foods your child readily accepts may grow out of your trying to be good to him. You aren't. Those tactics teach him to be incompetent with eating. It is better to do your feeding jobs, then let your child do his eating jobs (page 3). That shows him that you trust him to manage and that you trust him to grow up—with eating, as with all things.

Once you take control of the menu, how do you deal with a child who is skeptical about food?

- Let your child pick and choose from what you provide for the meal. He might eat only one or two foods.
- Don't force your child to eat—or even to taste—one food before he can have another.
- Don't try to please your child with every food. Settle for providing each eater—adults and children—with one or two foods they generally eat.
- Don't offer substitutes or short-order cook.
- When you introduce new foods, also offer something familiar that your child generally eats and can fill up on.
- Serve bread with every meal and let your child eat as much of it as he wants.
- Don't give choices on the main dish. Always putting out peanut butter or cereal with the meal tells your child, "I do not expect you to learn to eat new food."

Use "forbidden" food

At first, you will be on easy street. Your child won't know about high-fat, high-sugar, relatively low-nutrient foods such as sweets, chips, and sodas. But, sooner or later, someone will introduce them, and he is likely to eat these tasty, easy-to-like foods instantly and ask for more. These foods are part of our food world. Take the "specialness" out of them by having them regularly at family meals and snacks. He will eat as much as he is hungry for and then stop. If you try to avoid these foods, he is likely to eat a lot of them when he gets the chance.

- **Include chips or fries at mealtimes:** How often you do this is up to you. Arrange to have enough so you have some left over. Unlike sweets, fatty foods do not compete with other mealtime foods.
- **Have sweets for dessert (if you enjoy dessert), but limit everyone to one serving:** Put that one serving at each person's place. Let your child—or yourself—eat it at the beginning, during, or after the meal. Don't give seconds.
- **Offer unlimited sweets at snack-times:** Compensate at regular snack-times for mealtime sweets restriction. How often you do this is up to you. Offer milk and a plate of cookies. Have your child sit down and let him eat as many cookies and drink as much milk as he wants. At first, he will eat a lot, but then the newness will wear off and he won't eat so many.
- **Declare soda a grown-up drink:** It is. Your child will do best drinking milk or juice at meal- and snack-time. This will work until your child is 6 or 7 years old and discovers that other children drink soda!

Feeding stories: the toddler

You and your toddler will get into skirmishes—about feeding and about everything else. These stories about Oscar demonstrate some of the many ways your toddler will tempt you to do his jobs with feeding. Stay on your side of the division of responsibility, no matter how strongly your toddler invites you to cross it!

"I'm not hungry."

Oscar says "I'm not hungry" when his parents call him to dinner. At first, his parents say, "Oh dear, you *must* be hungry." Then they wise up: his being hungry is *his* business. Having a family meal is *their* business. So, they give him a five-minute warning. Then they say, "You don't have to eat, but come and keep us company while we eat." Sometimes Oscar eats happily for a while and then wants down. Sometimes he doesn't eat at all and wants down after a minute or two. At first, his parents keep him there in hopes that he will eat more. But he doesn't, and he makes such a commotion that they realize they have to let him down when he wants down.

"Now I'm hungry."

Oscar, having not eaten his meal, is back begging to sit on his daddy's lap and eat off his daddy's plate. When his daddy lets him, Oscar creates a commotion. So, his daddy says, "No, you have had your meal. That's it until snack time." Oscar tries his mother. She tells him the same thing. Oscar has a tantrum. His parents ignore him.

"Let's play."

Oscar, having more-or-less eaten his meal and been allowed to get down from the table, is back looking for attention while his parents try to enjoy their meal. They tell him to play, but he continues to pester. After the next meal, they wash Oscar up, clear away his dishes, put some toys not too far from the table, and spend a minute or two helping him get started playing. Then they go back to eating. They look at him from time to time while he plays and say or word or two. But they don't let him spoil their meal.

Avoid pressure

Pressure on children's eating *always* backfires. Keep in mind that all children are more-or-less picky about food. Trying to get a child to eat more than he wants makes him eat less. Trying to get him to eat less than he wants makes him eat more. Trying to get him to eat certain foods makes him avoid them. Trying to get him to be neat and tidy makes him messy. Putting up with negative behavior in hopes he will eat makes him behave badly but not eat. Here is what pressure looks like:

- Pressure can seem positive: Praising, reminding, bribing, rewarding, applauding, playing games, talking about nutrition, giving stickers, going on and on about how great the food is.
- Pressure can be negative: Restricting amounts or types of food; coaxing, punishing; shaming, criticizing, begging; withholding dessert, treats, or fun activities; physically forcing; threatening.
- Pressure can seem like good parenting: Reminding him to eat or to taste, making him eat his vegetables, warning him that he will be hungry, keeping after him to use his silverware or napkin, making special food, hiding vegetables in other foods, letting him eat whenever he wants to between meals.
- Pressure can be hard to detect: Ask yourself why you are doing something with feeding. Is it to get your child to eat more, less, or different food than he does on his own? If so, it is *pressure*.

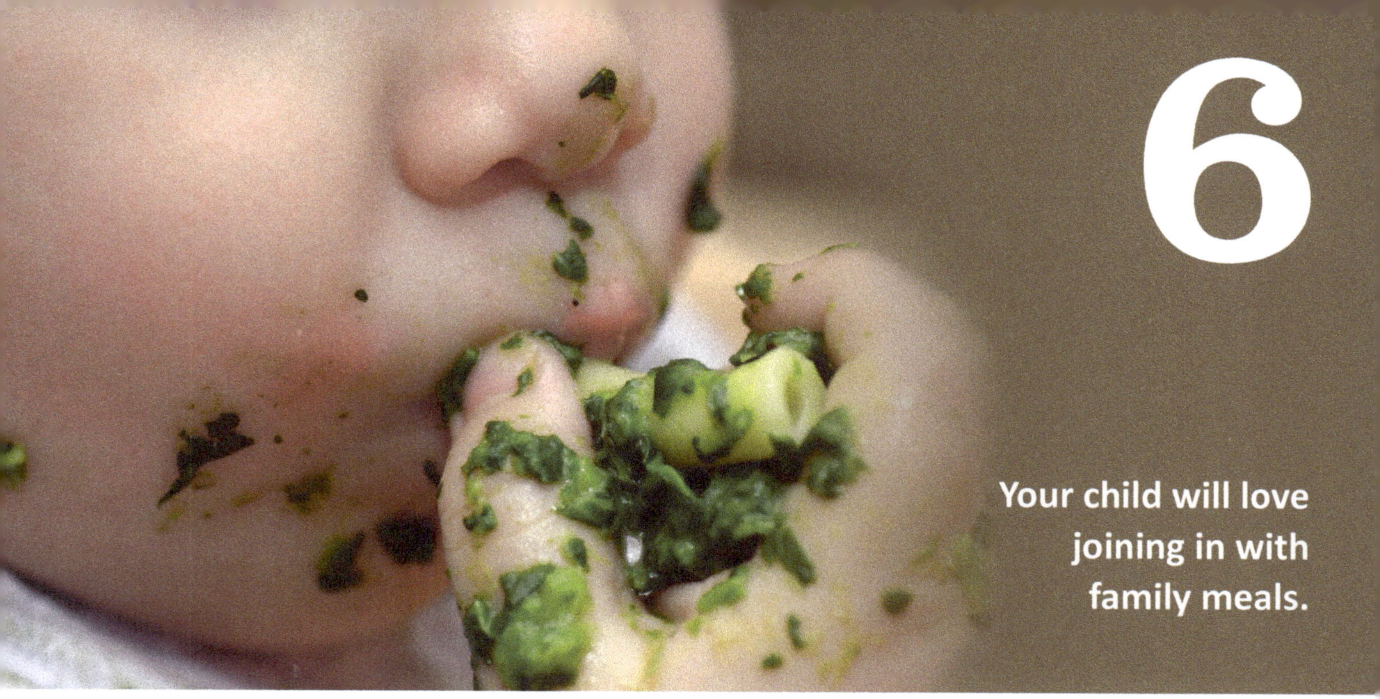

6. What to feed your child: step by step

Food selection for the older baby and almost-toddler is continuously in transition. You might move through the steps in 2 or 3 months, or it might take a year or more.

Steps 1 and 2 are for *learning,* not nourishment. Eating mushy and lumpy food is all new to your baby. She is getting used to getting fed from the spoon, learning how to do it, and feeling good about it, but not necessarily *eating.* Eating at the next stage depends on her getting used to the idea at this stage.

Steps 3 and 4 are for *nourishment* as well as for *learning.* When your child starts finger-feeding herself modified grown-up food, she will eat more solid food and less breastmilk or formula. Then she needs the nutrients from her solid food. Children who eat family food do better nutritionally than those who eat baby food.

For your child to eat well and behave well with food, use these strategies:

- ***Remember the division of responsibility in feeding:*** Do your jobs with *feeding* and let her do her jobs with *eating.*
- ***Start one new food at a time:*** Wait 3 or 4 days to give another new food. That lets you know whether a food gives your child a stomachache, diarrhea, skin rash, or wheezing.
- ***Give your child time and chances to learn to eat new food:*** After 10 or 20 tries (or more) in as many meals, your child will eat most foods.
- ***Seize the moment for including her in family mealtimes:*** During steps 3 and 4, your child's more-regular schedule and ability to feed herself makes it natural to include her in family meals.

Food Allergy

New evidence shows that you don't have to wait to start certain foods (such as eggs, fish, peanuts, or wheat) in order to avoid allergies. In fact, starting them earlier rather than later helps to prevent allergies. (If you have a lot of family allergies, talk with your doctor, especially about adding peanuts.) Add eggs, fish, wheat, and peanuts as your child gets developmentally ready, right along with other food. Don't rush, either. While some advice says to start allergenic foods by "4 to 6 months," you can safely wait until your child is developmentally ready to eat solid foods (page 20).

Step 1: mushy food you feed from the spoon

- ***Keep on nipple-feeding:*** Breastmilk or formula continues to be your child's most important source of nutrition until she is well established on grown-up food at step 4.
- ***Iron-fortified baby cereal mixed with breastmilk or formula:*** This is the best first solid food. To start, make the cereal about as thick as yogurt. Offer cereal once a day for the first few weeks and work up to offering it twice a day. Many parents feed only baby cereal at step 1 and wait to introduce fruits and vegetables in step 2.
- ***Finely mashed fruits and vegetables:*** If you prefer, you may start with pureed soft or cooked fruits and vegetables. These can be thoroughly fork-mashed, blended, baby-food-grinder prepared, or purchased as jarred baby food.

Step 2: thicker, lumpier food

Once your child learns to eat step 1 food, increase the thickness and lumpiness of the food. Lumps teach her to use her tongue to push food between her jaws where she mashes it. Some babies finger-feed themselves very thick food.

- ***Breastmilk or formula:*** Breastmilk or formula is still important. Along with her solid feedings, you may offer breastmilk or formula from a cup rather than from the nipple.
- ***Water:*** Offer your baby drinks of water from a cup. After she gets up from sleeping is a good time. You are checking to see if she is thirsty, not trying to get her to drink it.
- ***Thicker, lumpy, iron-fortified baby cereal:*** As time goes on, gradually make the cereal thicker and even lumpy. Thicken it still more to turn it into a finger food. Thicken other food with cereal to make it into finger food.
- ***Coarsely mashed fruits and vegetables:*** Some fruits can be raw, such as bananas, peaches, pears, mango, or melon. Cook tough or crisp fruits and vegetables, or use canned or frozen fruits and vegetables.
- ***Other soft food:*** Mashed potatoes, refried beans, sticky rice, cut up noodles.
- ***"Toddler" food from the store:*** All commercial baby food is completely smooth except for "toddler" food, which has step 2 texture. *Real* toddler food is *Step 4: modified grown-up food and drinks* (page 32).

Weaning starts with the first solid food

Weaning doesn't have to be hard or traumatic. It goes best when it is a gradual process of replacing nipple-feeding with solid food and drinking from a cup.

- Don't offer nipple-feeding before or along with the meal. Instead, offer breastmilk or formula in a cup.
- Let her skip her nipple-feeding afterward. She may eat so much she isn't interested!
- Work away from feeding on demand. Work toward offering nipple-feeding only for snacks, at set times between meals. Later, she will eat more "big-girl" snacks.
- Don't worry if at first her formula or breastmilk intake drops off. She will drink more when she gets better with the cup.

Step 3: finger food

A finger food is anything that sticks together long enough to get it from the high-chair tray to the mouth. Finger food teaches your child to use her tongue to push food between her jaws where she mashes it before she swallows. She will gag—that is all part of learning. See *Don't panic about gagging, but avoid choking* (page 21).

Finger foods can be small, soft pieces of the same foods you eat. Children who eat family food at family meals do better nutritionally than those who eat commercial baby food.

- ***Breastmilk or formula in a cup:*** Nipple-feeding is still all right for snacks until she is ready for "big-girl snacks." See *Weaning starts with the first solid food* on the previous page.
- ***Water in a cup:*** Offer water occasionally to check whether your child is thirsty, but don't get pushy with water. Your child knows how much water she needs.
- ***Cut-up raw soft fruit:*** Your child can gum and swallow bananas, peaches, pears, mango, melons, berries, and other soft fruit.
- ***Cut-up cooked vegetables, fruits, and casseroles:*** These are soft and moist and easy for your child to gum and swallow.
- ***Cheese, tender chopped meats:*** Have meat be tender and slice it across the grain into small pieces. Read the label on cheese to make sure it is made with pasteurized milk.
- ***Breakfast cereal:*** Cheerios, Corn Chex, Rice Chex, and Kix or their store brands are easy to pick up and gum. They also break down easily in saliva.
- ***Small pieces of bread or crackers:*** Try bread squares, toast strips, soft tortilla strips, graham crackers, and soda crackers.
- ***Adapt or avoid foods that can cause choking.*** Quarter grapes. Halve hot dogs the long way. Cut meat up finely. Don't give nuts, raw carrots, hard candy, jelly beans, and gum drops. Spread peanut butter thinly. Too-thick peanut butter can get stuck in her mouth and throat and make her choke.

Start offering sit-down, "big-girl" snacks

Snacks are little meals. They are not food handouts or treats. Your child's stomach is small, and her energy needs are high. To do well, she needs to eat every 2 or 3 hours.

Any food you have for meals works as a snack. Include two or three foods. To last a while, a snack needs to include protein, fat, and carbohydrate. Here are some examples:

- Bread or crackers with cheese or cheese spread and milk or fruit juice
- Cereal and whole or 2 percent milk
- Fresh or canned fruit with cheese or whole or 2 percent milk or whole-milk yogurt
- A fruit smoothie made of whole or 2 percent milk blended with fruit
- Vegetables, dip, and whole or 2 percent milk
- Cookies and whole or 2 percent milk

When meals are a long time apart, have two snacks: a long-lasting one early and a short-acting one (fruit, juice, crackers, frozen peas—think of it as an appetizer) to tide her over for dinner. But make it *a sit-down snack*. Don't allow your child to eat on the run or eat along with other activities.

Step 4: modified grown-up food and drinks

A child who can chew and swallow and use her fingers to pick up food is ready to eat most of the foods that you eat. Offer all the finger foods you added in step 3. Also offer any soft, easy-to-chew, cut-up food that you eat. *Don't panic about gagging, but avoid choking* (page 21). Offer milk in a cup (an open cup is better for learning than a sippy cup).

- ***Cut-up soft foods***: Spaghetti and other pasta dishes, burritos, potatoes (scalloped, mashed, baked with sour cream or butter).
- ***Toasts and sandwiches:*** Cheese toast or grilled cheese. Shaved turkey, ham, or bologna and cheese. Thinly spread peanut butter.
- ***Meat and other protein foods:*** Fried, baked, or roasted chicken (tender and finely cut); roasts or chops (tender and finely cut); fish (remove all the bones); other proteins such as eggs, dried beans, peas, lentils, and soy-based meat substitutes.
- ***Fast food:*** Take-out or frozen pizza cut into bite-sized pieces and cooled down, burgers cut into strips, cut-up chicken nuggets, burritos, soft French fries.
- ***Ethnic food:*** Ask parents from other cultures what they feed their young children; especially ask what they do about spicy food.

When and how to give whole milk

For bottles, continue to use breastmilk or formula. **Never** serve unpasteurized milk of any kind at any age. In the cup, *along with meals and snacks*, you may change to whole *pasteurized* milk ***if***

- Your child drinks the pasteurized milk ***from a cup, and***
- She is well-established on grown-up food, ***and***
- She eats at least 2 or 3 ounces of solid food at each meal or snack.

If your child was prematurely born or had a slow start for any other reason, it is best to keep her on breastmilk or formula for a while longer. She needs the nutrition, and her digestive tract needs longer to mature.

When and how to give juice

Your child gets her vitamins and minerals from breastmilk or formula, so she does not need juice until she starts drinking regular milk. Give juice in a cup, not in the bottle. That helps keep her from getting stuck on the bottle. Serve only 100 percent fruit or vegetable juice. Canned, bottled, or powdered fruit *drinks* do not give as much nutrition as fruit *juice*. Serve juice only at mealtime or snack-time, not in-between times. Don't let your child carry around a sippy cup or bottle containing anything except water.

When and how to give sweets and fatty snacks

Before long, someone will introduce your child to cookies, candy, potato chips, and other salty fried snacks. Because high-sugar, high-fat foods are easy to like, she will eat them instantly and beg for them soon after. Do not despair. Your child's energy needs are high and her stomach is small, so she benefits from eating some high-sugar, high-fat foods. It is impossible to avoid these foods, so don't try. Instead, learn to make wise use of them. See page 27, "Use forbidden food".

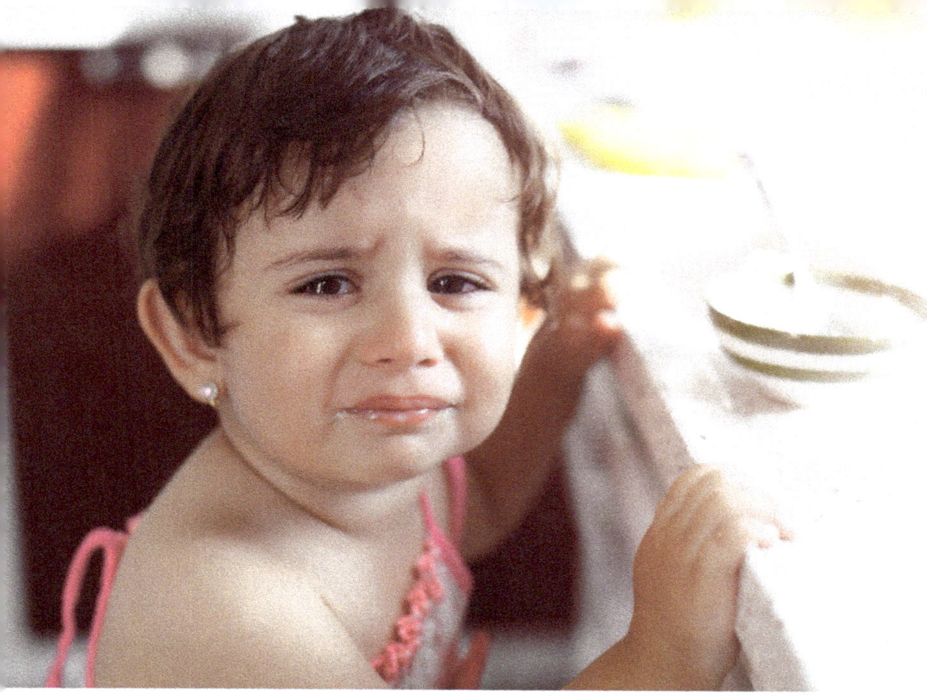

7

Maintain structure and avoid pressure.

7. Solve feeding problems

"My toddler will not eat at mealtime and then begs for food."

Don't attempt to solve the problem by trying to get your child to eat more at mealtime. He won't. Instead, support him in eating as well as he can at mealtime by being careful to follow the division of responsibility. Resign yourself to the fact that *The toddler's eating is quirky* (page 26). *Avoid common feeding mistakes* (page 26).

Don't, say, "Why didn't you eat more? See what I told you—you didn't eat enough, and now you are hungry. Oh, all right, what do you want? But next time you have to eat!"

Instead, say, "The meal is over, but snack-time is coming soon. You can eat then." Then stick to what you say. He is learning that "no" means "no." He may pitch a fit. Ignore him. When he gets done yelling and kicking, the answer is still "no." After 2 or 3 days, he will learn to eat (in a toddler's typically quirky way) at meal- and snack-time.

"Isn't that a little harsh?" parents ask. "After all, he is so little and it is only one little cookie. What if I offered him whole-wheat crackers instead? Why make such a big deal over it?"

Sorry, it is a big deal. *Your child depends on you to set the limit*. If you give in to his food-begging, the list of foods he eats will become shorter and shorter, and his behavior at meals will get worse and worse. Not only that, it scares him to get the upper hand with you.

Your child needs to learn that being included in family meals is special. It is special because he gets to be part of the family and because he gets to eat. Teach him that to be there, he has to behave nicely and cope with the food you provide for the meal. Behave nicely yourself by not interfering with his eating jobs.

Set and follow a schedule of meals and snacks every 2 or 3 hours. Always offer bread (or something like it). If all he eats is the bread, that is okay. If he eats a *lot* of bread, that is still okay. But don't get out the peanut butter or the cereal. Those are different meals and count as short-order cooking. It tells your child, "I do not trust you to learn to eat the food I eat."

If the struggles go on, take another look at *Have family-friendly meals* (page 24) and *Avoid pressure* (page 28).

“My child is too small or does not eat enough.”

Follow the division of responsibility. Your child will eat and grow best when you concentrate on the *quality* of the feeding rather than the *quantity* of food. The research is clear: Children eat less when parents try to get them to eat.

Even before she is ready to eat family meals, show your child what eating is all about. Follow the division of responsibility. *Have family-friendly meals* (page 24). *Avoid pressure* (page 28).

- Do your jobs with *feeding,* and trust your child to do her jobs with *eating* (page 4). Don’t try to get her to eat a certain amount. Don’t praise your child for eating or scold her for not eating.
- *Trust your child to grow in the best way* (page 4). Don’t try to get her to be bigger than nature intended for her.

Protect yourself from interference. Often children are labeled *too small* or even *failure to thrive* when their growth is below the third or even the fifth percentile. But if your child grows consistently at *any* level—that is, if her weight and height are at or near the same percentiles at each doctor visit—then she is growing well and is just small. Trying to change her natural growth pattern will make you both miserable and is unlikely to succeed.

Trying to change your child’s natural growth pattern will make you both miserable and is unlikely to succeed.

Crossing growth percentiles. A child’s growth can gradually go up if she was small to begin with. But it is concerning for a child’s growth to *abruptly* go up or down. To let your child grow in the way that is right for her, follow the division of responsibility. *Get help if you are stuck* (page 40), and *Consider a feeding relationship collaboration* (page 40). Read *Child of Mine: Feeding with Love and Good Sense.*

Hold steady with feeding, even in the face of illness

My son Jacob was born with a heart defect and needed surgery. The doctors wanted him to be a certain weight before they would operate. But Jacob’s heart defect made it hard for him to eat. He could not breathe well, and he did not have much energy. We concentrated his formula, but he still wore out before he ate much. Even though the doctors told me to get a certain amount into him, I knew better than to force him. But it was so *hard.* Some days he would eat more, and I would think, “That’s it! He has finally turned a corner!” But the next day he would not eat much at all, and my spirits would take a nose-dive. It helped *so much* when the dietitian showed me a graph of a well baby’s formula intake. It was up and down, just like Jacob’s! After that, I trusted Jacob more, and feeding went better. Before long, he gained enough weight to have his surgery.

"My child is too big or eats too much."

Many infants and toddlers are chubby. In spite of common opinion, the fat baby or toddler is no more likely to grow up fat than the thin one. Maintaining the division of responsibility with a large child is not easy in today's fat-phobic world. If you worry about your own weight, it is even harder. But it works.

Compare your child to himself. Pay attention to how your child grows *over time*. Is he growing *consistently*? Even if his weight is high, he is growing well if his weight is at or near the same percentile at each doctor visit. Remember:

- Follow the division of responsibility. Don't withhold food. He will get scared and eat too much when he gets the chance. Even big children are entitled to eat as much as they are hungry for.
- *Follow the division of responsiblity with activity* (page 5). Don't try to get your child to be more active in order to slim him down. He will lose his joy of moving and stop doing it when he gets the chance.
- *Trust your child to grow in the best way* (page 4). Don't try to get him to be smaller or slimmer than nature intended for him.

Rose slimmed down

Rose's weight was over the ninety-fifth percentile when she was born and she got bigger and bigger, even though I tried to keep her from eating as much as she wanted. When she was 11 months old, someone gave me a copy of *Child of Mine.* I studied it carefully and started following a division of responsibility. I let Rose eat as much as she wanted at meals and snacks. She ate so much, and I was so anxious! But within a couple of weeks, her eating settled down. She ever-so-gradually slimmed down, and by the time she was 4 she was back on the growth chart, and by age 7 her BMI was down to the eighty-fifth percentile. Now she is a teenager, and her BMI is at about the seventy-fifth percentile. She enjoys eating, is active and coordinated, and is comfortable with her body.

Don't let anyone tell you your child is too fat. Your infant or child who grows at the eighty-fifth percentile (weight or BMI) may be labeled *overweight.* Your infant or child who grows at the ninety-fifth percentile may be labeled *obese*. Ignore such labels. Studies show that, at every weight level, children gain too much weight when parents see them as being "overweight." Why? Parents of "too fat" children are likely to try to get them to eat less. Which backfires: Restricted children eat more and get heavier. Not only that, but when such "too-fat" children get older, they feel bad about their bodies and try to diet to lose weight. Which also backfires.

Crossing growth percentiles. A child's growth can gradually go down to a lower percentile if he was big to begin with. But it is concerning if growth abruptly goes down—or up. To let your child grow in the way that is right for him, follow the division of responsibility. *Get help if you are stuck* (page 40), and *Consider a feeding relationship collaboration* (page 40). Read *Your Child's Weight: Helping without Harming.*

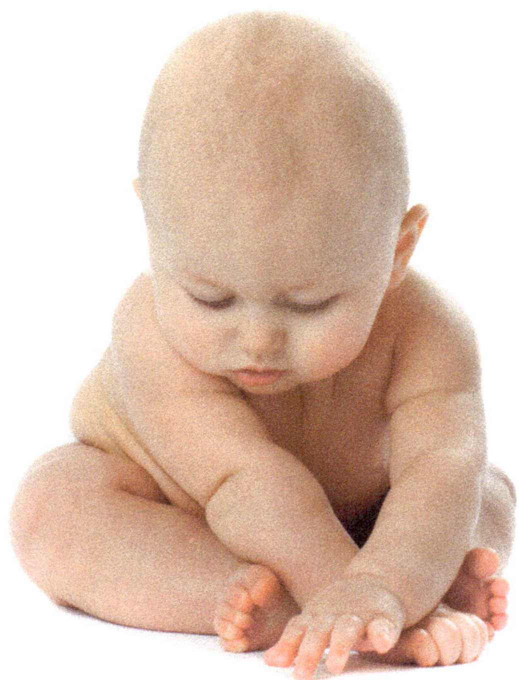

"My child is a picky eater."

All children are more or less picky about food. Some children are finicky. Picky is normal; finicky is a problem.

What *picky* looks like: Your child likes to come to family meals and behaves well there. She eats one or two food items, ignores food she does not want to eat, and eats a food one day but not the next. She watches you eat new food (or food she *thinks* is new), touches it, puts it in her mouth, and takes it back out again. You might serve a food at as many as 15 or 20 meals or *countless* meals before she eats it.

What *finicky* looks like: Your child does not want to come to family meals and behaves poorly there. She gets upset if she sees anything but the short list of foods that she eats. Even when those foods are there, she often will not eat. You get aggravated and find yourself trying to get her to eat.

Finicky eaters can be born or made, or both. Some children are sensitive to new tastes or textures—or to anything new, period. Someone may even say your child has "sensory issues." But even children with "sensory issues" push themselves along to learn as long as they have chances to learn and *no pressure*. A finicky eater is *made* by not having chances to get comfortable with unfamiliar food and by being pressured to eat. Keep in mind that short-order cooking puts pressure on a child to eat the food you made especially for her.

The finicky eater needs chances to learn and no pressure.

How to address finicky eating: You can't get your child to eat, but you do need to teach her to behave nicely at mealtime. She wants to please you, but it is simply beyond her to eat what you want her to eat. You can, however, change your expectations and stop pressuring her to eat. Show her how to please you by behaving nicely at mealtime. When she is comfortable and behaves well at mealtime and you *Avoid pressure* (page 28), she will ever-so-gradually push herself along to learn to eat new foods. Don't hold your breath—it could take *years*.

Teach your child to behave well at mealtime

- Have mealtime be pleasant. Include her in conversation.
- Be sure to include one or two foods she generally eats.
- Teach her to say "yes, please" and "no, thank you." Don't let her say *"yuck!"*
- Give her an out: "You don't have to eat if you don't want." Give her encouragement: "You can find something to eat."
- Have her leave the meal if she behaves badly. Don't let her have food again until the next meal or snack.
- Let her leave the meal when she is finished. Don't keep her there in hopes she will eat more. She won't.

Remember, follow the division of responsibility, *Have family-friendly meals* (page 24), and *Avoid pressure* (page 28).

Your child will not be picky forever

My kids were extremely picky eaters as toddlers and young children, but we stayed the course with the division of responsibility. It took many years, but we got there. I distinctly remember the first time my son asked us to pass the broccoli. We did so without any fanfare—as if he asked for it every night of his life—but inside I was jumping for joy. The division of responsibility truly does work for the long term. My kids are now teenagers, and it gives me great satisfaction to see them eat a wide variety of food with gusto.

"My child will not eat vegetables (or fruits)... and I don't enjoy them much either!"

While vegetables and fruits are good for you, they are not worth fighting about. When you follow the division of responsibility in feeding and enjoy fruits and vegetables yourself, your child will eventually enjoy them, too. Don't force your child or yourself to eat them. You cannot fake it. Studies show that parents who eat—and enjoy—vegetables have children who eat—and enjoy—vegetables. Parents who eat but *do not* enjoy vegetables have children who do not eat vegetables and do not enjoy them. If you want your child to enjoy fruits and vegetables, you need to enjoy them yourself.

How you and your child can learn to enjoy fruits and vegetables:

- **Apply feeding principles to including vegetables:** Follow the division of responsibility, *Have family-friendly meals* (page 24), and *Avoid pressure* (page 28).
- **Sneak up on them:** Your child looks but does not taste, tastes but does not swallow. You can look in the grocery store. Buy a little, prepare a little, taste a little, throw away a little. Take your time.
- **Try, try, try again:** Plan on 10 to 20 tries in as many meals—or even more— to learn to eat a new food. Better still, stop counting.
- **Don't get pushy:** Everybody learns better with an out. You can decide not to eat it even if you bought it and cooked it.
- **Prepare vegetables and fruits the way you enjoy them:** They can be raw, cooked until they are just tender, or cooked until they are really soft.
- **Make them taste good:** Add sugar to fruits. Bake fruit pies or cobbler. Dress vegetables up with butter, cream, oil, bacon, fat back, white sauce, cheese sauce, herbs and spices, or brown sugar. Put vegetables in soups and stews.
- **Don't trick your child into eating vegetables:** Your child will catch on and not trust you.
- **Know that some vegetables are hard to enjoy:** People who are *super-tasters* say broccoli, cabbage, cauliflower, and some greens taste strong and even bitter. Tone them down with butter, salt, or sauces.

Don't get pushy. Everybody learns better with an out.

Your child will eat vegetables . . . someday

When Kjerstin was little, she would not touch a vegetable. I prepared family meals, and I always included nicely prepared vegetables. I figured that if she did not want to eat vegetables, I could not make her. I was surprised when I heard how upset other moms were about their kids not eating vegetables. They were actually getting into fights about it! One mom was proud of putting zucchini in the hamburger patties and beets in the brownies. I was not willing to trick Kjerstin. I knew sooner or later she would catch on, and then she would not trust me. When Kjerstin was around 11 years old, she seemed to notice that she was missing out, and she started eating—and enjoying—vegetables. She did it all on her own. I am sure if we had tricked or forced her, she would never have done it.

"My child will not drink milk."

Children depend on milk for calcium, vitamin D, and protein. Today's children who drink soda instead of milk have smaller bones and more broken bones. See *When and how to give whole milk* (page 32). Children's milk intake often drops right after they are weaned from the breast or bottle. Then, after a few months, it gradually goes back up again.

Offer milk in the best way: You cannot make your child drink milk. But you can do a good job with feeding. That will encourage her to go back to drinking milk. Here is how:

- **Drink milk yourself:** If you drink milk, your child will think, "That is what grown-ups drink." Even if she does not drink milk today, she will someday.
- **Even if milk gives you stomachaches or diarrhea, it probably will not bother your toddler:** Children do not become lactose intolerant until they are 4 or 5 years old.
- **You still might be able to drink a little milk:** You might tolerate a small glass of whole or 2% milk with meals. Consider a soy, rice, oat, or other milk-substitute beverage. Compare labels to see if the substitute has as much protein, calcium, and vitamin D as milk.
- **If you cannot drink milk, drink water:** Do not have soda, juice, Kool-Aid, sweet tea, or other sweet drinks if you want your child to drink milk. At mealtime, let her have water as well as milk.
- **Don't get pushy:** Put a small glass of milk at your child's place, and let her drink it or not. Don't remind her to drink it (that is pressure). She knows it is there.
- **Serve other food that has calcium in it:** That might be cheese, yogurt, or orange juice with calcium. See *When and how to give juice* (page 32).
- **Don't go overboard with flavored milks:** Chocolate or strawberry milk is fine once in a while. But regularly flavoring milk to get it into your child is pressure, and pressure backfires.

Adrian was on-again, off-again with milk

I distinctly remember the day Adrian went cold turkey on milk. I wailed, "But you love milk!" and he just looked at me. So I stopped saying anything. At every meal, I put a small glass of milk at his place. He didn't make a fuss—he just ignored it. I frankly don't remember how long it was before he started drinking it again. I didn't say anything then, either. Now at age 11 he drinks a lot of milk. And eats a lot of everything else!

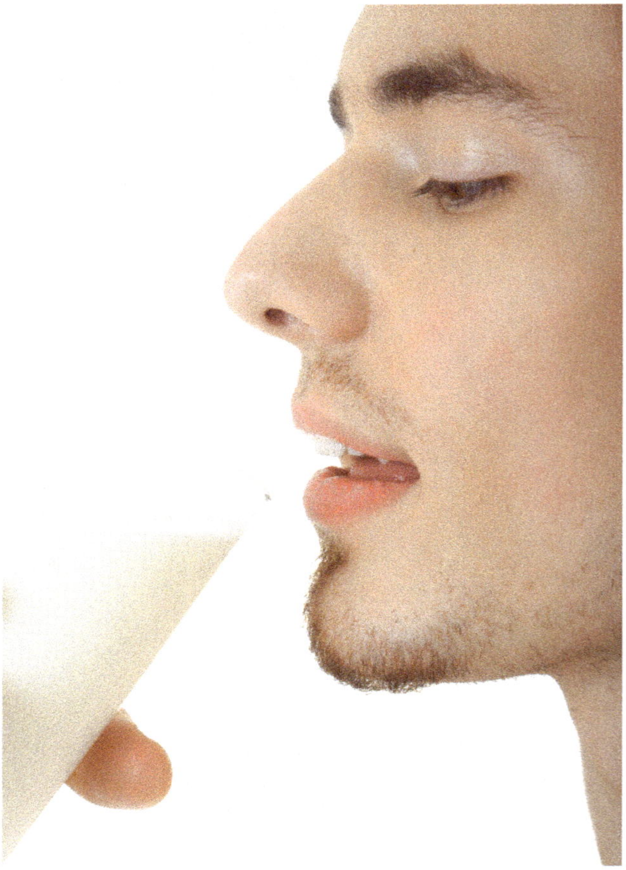

Your child will drink milk if you do.

"My child has special needs."

The biggest problem with feeding your "child with special needs" is that any diagnosis undermines your trust in your child to eat. That need not be. At the same time as you must be attentive to medical, developmental, and oral-motor issues, your child is more *child* than *special needs*. He *wants* to grow up, and he *will* grow up to the very best of his ability. Most of his feeding issues are the same as those of any other child. His stages in feeding look the same; they just come along more slowly. His challenges at each stage are the same; he just works harder and longer to master them. His eating quirks are the same; it is just hard for you to sort out the "child" in these quirks from the "special." It really doesn't matter.

The division of responsibility in feeding works for children with special needs.

Trust your child with special needs

- Trust is the foundation of good parenting with feeding: trusting yourself; trusting your child.
- Your child wants to eat, and he wants to grow up with eating.
- He eats best (most, greatest variety) when you give him opportunities to learn and *no pressure*.
- At first, your child with special needs is likely to be medically fragile.
- Fragile children scare everyone, even experienced health professionals.
- Scared people tend to put pressure on feeding.
- Putting pressure on feeding takes away trust and takes away your child's desire to grow up with eating.
- See *Consider a feeding relationship collaboration* (next page).

Arthur wanted to eat

Arthur was born a few weeks early. Nipple-feeding was challenging, but we worked it out. The trouble began when he started solid foods. Looking back, I can see that Arthur was slow to learn, and I got scared and put pressure on him to eat. He was reluctant to eat solid foods, gagged on finger food, and refused anything moist. By age two-and-a-half, he ate very few foods and put up a fuss when I tried to get him to the table. He even gagged or vomited when he watched others eat!

Arthur's doctor sent us to a feeding clinic. We were told that Arthur's eating issues were behavioral and that a child with a feeding problem would starve rather than eat foods beyond his comfort level. They held food in front of Arthur until he gave in and ate it, praised him when he ate, ignored him when he didn't, gave him stickers when he ate, and time-outs when he didn't. We realized they were force-feeding him, but we went along when they taught us the same routine for at home. Feeding was awful, but Arthur ate more food and a greater variety. It did not last. After a year, he rebelled against the force-feeding, and his eating went back to what it was when we first went to the feeding clinic.

So, I gathered my courage, went back to the division of responsibility, and followed it to the letter. This time, I was careful to avoid pressure in every way. Arthur ate little and gagged watching us eat. It was agony for me, and I questioned my decision daily. After a couple of weeks, he began to come willingly to the table. After that, he gradually ate more, and he began experimenting with new food.

Instead of piling on more pressure, I wish the feeding clinic had helped me stop the pressure and trust Arthur to eat. Being slow to learn was just his way. All along, Arthur wanted to eat. Now that I let him take his time, he pushes himself along to eat foods beyond his comfort level.

Get help if you are stuck

Though no fault of your own or anyone else, your child may have developed an established feeding problem. The problem has a history. Your child may have had temperamental, medical, and/or developmental issues that created negative feeding patterns. Such patterns attract negative advice that doesn't work or that makes matters worse.

How to tell you are stuck

- Your child's growth veers upward or downward abruptly.
- You are making no progress getting on your child's wavelength with feeding.
- Your struggles with feeding go on and on.
- You cannot maintain the division of responsibility in feeding.

Consider an assessment

An assessment will restore your trust in your child to do her part with feeding. It is normal for your child to eat and grow normally. What got (or continues to get) in the way of her natural eating competence? To find answers, enlist the help of a professional who is expert in applying the division of responsibility in feeding. With your adviser, begin by doing an assessment that considers your child's medical history and growth pattern from birth, your past and present feeding relationship, your relationship as a whole, the structure of family meals and snacks, and your child's nutrition.

Consider a feeding relationship collaboration

Most feeding clinics use behavioral interventions that cross the lines of the division of responsibility and focus on getting children to eat. Instead, look for a professional who thoroughly understands the division of responsibility in feeding. It is best to have in-person help from a local professional who has been mentored and trained by the Ellyn Satter Institute (ESI). Because professionals who fully understand and properly apply the Satter Eating Competence Model and the Satter division of responsibility in feeding are currently a select group, ESI offers virtual coaching services. ESI faculty members and associates can connect with you by computer to help you find a successful and rewarding way to feed your child. You can find ESI coaching at https://www.ellynsatterinstitute.org. Your coach will help you to:

- Follow the division of responsibility.
- Feed in a developmentally appropriate fashion (page 19).
- At each stage, provide your child with opportunities to learn; then wait, wait, and wait some more.
- Know the signs of progress. Your child will relax at feeding time, enjoy that time with you, and forget about eating between times.
- Be entirely neutral, both in the way you present food and in the way you react to your child's eating and not eating. Be extremely careful to *Avoid pressure* (page 28).
- Expect that your child will not do, not do, not do, then do.
- Be prepared for the long haul. Like other children, your child may be a teenager before some of his eating problems are resolved.
- Do problem solving when your child's eating relapses. Chances are, structure is eroding or pressure is creeping in.
- Seek out special services if your child needs them. He may benefit from occupational therapy to improve his chewing and swallowing. On the other hand, he may provide his own occupational therapy by pushing himself along to learn to chew and swallow.

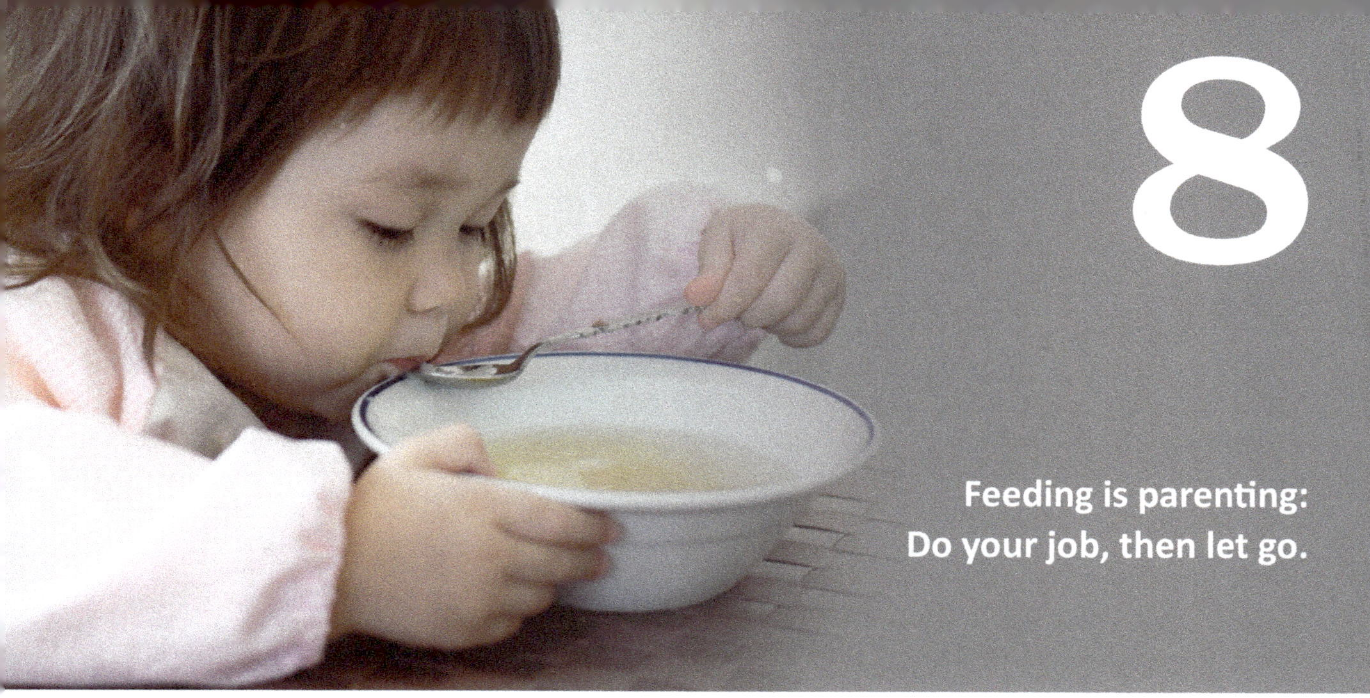

8. What you have learned

When you follow the division of responsibility in feeding, your child will be a good eater.

It is all about control. You can control some things; you cannot control others. You can control what your child is offered to eat. You cannot control whether she eats it, how much she eats, and how she grows. Feeding is parenting in all ways. You have to do your jobs, but then you have to let go.

Your child knows how much (or little) to eat. From birth, your child knows how much to eat and how to grow. Your job is to read her signs and do what works best for her at her stage of development. If your child's weight is following a consistent percentile on her growth chart, she is growing just fine.

Your child will grow up to eat the food you eat. On some level, your child thinks, "I will eat that someday." And she pushes herself along as fast as she can to do just that.

Provide, don't deprive, and don't pressure. Trust your child to grow up to be the size and shape that nature intended. Feel good about the child you *have*, not the one you *thought* you might have.

Emma taught me how to eat

My eating problems grew out of not having proper meals, which grew out of dieting. It helped a lot when we decided, on our daughter Emma's behalf, to eat at the table every night. I discovered I can go to the table hungry and eat until I have enough! Trying to fill up on vegetables to save calories turned me off on them, but since Emma and her daddy genuinely enjoy them, I find I can get back to enjoying them too! I felt that I had no stopping place, especially with sweets. Emma showed me what having a stopping place is all about. She loves sweets, so at meals we regularly offer her a child-sized dessert and at occasional snacks a many sweets as she wants. Emma eats her dessert, then eats the rest of her food. At snacks, she eats a couple of cookies and is done.

What is next

Now you know most of what you need to know about feeding, and your child has become a competent eater. What you have learned in this booklet will guide you for the rest of your years of parenting with feeding. You have established and maintained a division of responsibility in feeding. In the process of navigating your child's many changes in these first 2 years, you have learned to trust your child to do his part with eating and growing. From now on, the task is for you to remain a good feeder and for your child to remain a good eater.

Keep these principles in mind for feeding your child in all the stages to come. As your child gets older, consider reading the other booklets in this series, pictured on the back cover. They address following the division of responsibility in feeding the preschooler, school-aged child, and adolescent. For more in-depth information about the why as well as the how of feeding, consider reading *Child of Mine: Feeding with Love and Good Sense* as well as *Your Child's Weight: Helping without Harming*. For help with planning and preparing family meals, read "How to Cook" in *Secrets of Feeding a Healthy Family*.

Your child can teach you about your own eating

- Let your child show you what relaxed and joyful eating is all about. Keep your mouth shut and your fingers crossed and the look of surprise (or panic) off your face.
- Reassure *yourself* you will be fed and that you can have food that you enjoy.
- Work your way through booklet five in this series, *Feeding* Yourself *with Love and Good Sense*, available at *www.EllynSatterInstitute.org*.
- Read more. Click on *How to Eat* on *www.EllynSatterInstitute.org.* Read "Part 1, How to Eat" in *Secrets of Feeding a Healthy Family.*

Reach out to others

Has this booklet been helpful to you? Would you like others to be helped to feel confident and relaxed about feeding? Here is what you can do:

- Tell a friend about it. Buy them a copy.
- Tell your health professional about it. Encourage them to purchase in bulk for their office by contacting *support@ellynsatterinstitute.org*.
- Tell your nutrition, health, or wellness teacher about it. Encourage them to purchase in bulk and use it as part of their curriculum.
- Talk about it on social media. Share your experience of becoming successful and joyful with feeding and confidently addressing your child's eating problems.

www.ingramcontent.com/pod-product-compliance
Lightning Source LLC
Jackson TN
JSHW041231150626
103893JS00006B/12
9781971847054